HOW TO LIVE WITH SICKLE CELL:

Sickle Cell and I

Tola Dehinde

Dedication & Thanksgiving

I dedicate this book to everyone born with Sickle Cell Disorder and all care-givers, who come in various forms (family members, loved ones and friends).

I particularly want to thank my sister friends both near and far, the one who would come and pick me up before going to work and drop me at the hospital first thing in the mornings when I am sick and need to go to the day clinic. I want to thank my sister friends who would cook for me and bring or send the food over. I want to thank those who would pray for me amongst so many other acts of kindness.

I would like to thank those who would phone me, checking on me via texts and all. I thank you all because we have a system that works for me, some of you know talking when I am in so much pain can be draining for me and so you send me prayers that I read or voice notes that I listen to.

I also want to thank my brothers in Christ, who reach out to me from time to time, especially the one who lives in Ghana (you know who you are), I thank you all.

I would also like to thank my siblings, Yetunde, Baba and Segun, who endured lots of sleepless nights and interrupted programmes whenever I was sick as we grew up. You guys never moaned, thank you!

Most of all, I would like to thank my parents, Mr & Mrs Dehinde; especially my mother for her motherly love and care whenever I am sick till date.

TABLE OF CONTENTS

DEFINITION OF SICKLE CELL ANEMIA

Sickle cell disorder (SCD) is a disease of the haemoglobin in the red blood cells.

Haemoglobin is the substance in red blood cells that is responsible for the colour of the cell and for carrying oxygen around the body.

People with sickle cell disorder are born with the condition, it is not contagious. It can only be inherited from both parents each having passed on the gene for sickle cell.

What are sickle cell anemia and SCD?

Sickle cell anemia (SCA) is a serious condition which is inherited (genetic). It affects the red blood cells in the blood. With SCA, the red blood cells have a tendency to go out of shape and become sickle-shaped (like a crescent moon) – instead of their normal doughnut/disc shape. This can cause various problems such as episodes of pain, infections and various complications.

Indeed, the terms sickle cell anemia and sickle cell disease or sickle cell disorder are often used interchangeably. However, there are various other disorders that are classified as subtypes of SCD with each having a slightly different genetic makeup. Examples are sickle cell/beta thalassemia and sickle cell/HbC.

The main symptoms of sickle cell disorder are anemia and episodes of severe pain. The pain occurs when the cells change shape after oxygen has been released. The red blood cells then stick together, causing blockages in the small blood vessels. These painful episodes are treated with strong painkillers such as morphine to control the pain.

People with sickle cell are at risk of further complications such as stroke, acute chest syndrome, blindness, bone damage and priapism (a persistent, painful erection of the penis) etc.

Sickle cell disorder affects millions of people throughout the world and is particularly common among those whose ancestors came from sub-Saharan African; Spanish-speaking regions in the Western Hemisphere (South America, the Caribbean, and Central America).

It is also widely spread through the Middle East, Southeast Asia (India), and Mediterranean countries such as Turkey, Greece and Italy.

Sickle cell disease (SCD) is one of the most prevalent genetic disorders worldwide. Nigeria has the largest population of people living with SCD in the world with over 90,000 babies born in a year. According to the Sickle Cell Society, approximately 15,000 people in the UK have SCD.

Studies have reported a count of approximately 100,000 Americans being affected by this disease. It is also estimated that one in 500 US African American births is affected with SCD. In some parts of central Africa, as many as one person in 40 is born with the disease.

About 4 million people in West and Central Africa suffer from the disease; from 500,000 to 1 million people in South America.

Over time people with sickle cell can experience damage to organs such as the liver, kidney, lungs, heart and spleen. Death can also result from complications of the disorder. Treatment of sickle cell mostly focuses on managing the pain, preventing and treating complications.

The only possible cure for the disorder is bone marrow transplant but this is only possible for a limited number of affected individuals who have a suitable donor. A tablet called Hydroxyurea, can significantly reduce the number of painful crises.

Did you know?

SCD is inherited from both parents, sickle cell trait is inherited from one parent;

SCD can affect anyone, although it predominantly affects people from African and Caribbean; Mediterranean, Asia and the Middle East. *(There are other nationalities affected too).*

A simple blood test will tell whether you have SC trait or the disorder.

Children with SCD are at increased risk of stroke, the risk is highest between the ages of 2 -16.

Episode of pains may occur in SCD and is generally referred to as a crisis.

SICKLE CELL AND 6 TYPES OF SC CRISES

Did you know that there are six different types of crises that people with Sickle cell have to endure? The most common is vaso-occlusive but let us look through them all in detail:-

Vaso-occlusive crisis – is a painful sickle cell crisis (or vaso-occlusive crisis); it is the commonest manifestation of SCD and is characterized by recurrent episodes of acute, severe pain from tissue ischemia as a result of vasco-occlusion. Sickle cell anemia patients often experience episodes of acute pain that are caused by vaso-occlusive crisis (VOC).

Hemoglobin is a protein inside red blood cells and is responsible for transporting oxygen. Hemoglobin S molecules tend to stick together and form aggregates. These aggregates distort the shape of red blood cells, resulting in so-called sickle-shaped red blood cells. Hemoglobin S also damages the membrane of red blood cells, which makes them sticky. As a result, the cells tend to adhere to the inner lining of blood vessels. Sickle red blood cells also are stiffer than normal blood cells. The combination of these two characteristics is thought to promote the blockage of small blood vessels, which prevents oxygen supple to tissues and causes injury.

Patients with Sickle cell anemia may experience VOC several times per year. Pain is unpredictable and frequently occurs spontaneously but may be seen after infection, exposure to cold, dehydration or in uncommon situations after emotional stress, exercise or alcohol, often no precipitation cause can be found, as triggers of VOC are not entirely understood.

VOC crisis is responsible for around 90% of hospital admission and visits in patients with SCD. Legs, arms, back, chest and abdomen are often involved in VOC. VOC might cause leg ulcers, stroke, kidney insufficiency and spontaneous abortion.

Acute splenic sequestration (ASS) – Splenic sequestration is the enlargement of the spleen that can be life-threatening. There are 2 types of splenic sequestration in Sickle cell disease (acute and chronic). Chronic splenic sequestration may not cause problems and the doctor may choose to record the size of the spleen at each visit to make sure it is not getting any larger. ASS can happen when sickled red blood cells get trapped in the spleen, causing the spleen to enlarge.

Sickle cell disease affects the red blood cells causing them to sickle or become banana-shaped. The main purpose of red blood cells (RBCs) is to deliver oxygen to the body. Sickled RBCs stick together and slow the flow of oxygen to the tissues. When sickled RBCs are trapped in the spleen, the rest of the body does not get enough oxygen. If not treated, ASS, can cause the body to go into shock.

What then is the spleen? The spleen is an oval-shaped organ located on the left side of the body. It is protected by the ribcage. Functions of the spleen: it fights invading germs in the blood (the spleen contains infection-fighting white blood cells); it controls the level of blood cells (white blood cells, red blood cells and platelets); it filters the blood and removes any old or damaged red blood cells.

The immediate treatment is red blood cell transfusion as this provides the body with much needed oxygen to the cells and releases the sickled RBCs trapped in the spleen. The spleen reduces in size and the anemia is corrected.

The chances of having another episode of ASS are high. If the first episode was severed or if a second ASS occurs, the doctor may recommend splenectomy (removal of the spleen). A person can live without a spleen because other organs in the body perform the same function as the spleen. So, a person can have a healthy life without the spleen.

Infarctive crisis – Infarction (obstruction of the blood supply to an organ) of the bone marrow leads to release of inflammatory meditators which activate afferent nerve fibres resulting in severe generalized bone pain. Almost any bone may be involved and there is a tendency for the infarcts to become infected. Sometimes infection may occur.

Aplastic crisis (AC) is when the body does not make enough new Red Blood Cells to replace the ones that are already in the blood. Normally, the soft tissue at the centre of your bones, called bone marrow, constantly make new RBCs. These cells go into your blood supply and carry oxygen through the body. If you have SCD, your body needs to make a lot of new RBCs but during AC, the bone marrow stops making RBCs for a short time. This is called transient (temporary) AC. It normally lasts for 7-10 days; after which the bone marrow starts making RBCs again.

AC is usually caused by a virus. Parvovirus B19 is one of the most common causes. The virus causes the bone marrow to stop making a new RBCs for 7-10 days.

An AC is not a problem for most people, because normal RBCs last 90-120 days but it is a serious problem in people with SCD. Their RBCs only last 7-20 days and if the sickled cells stops making RBCs for a few days, they can get severed anemia.

Haemolytic crisis (HC) is an acute drop in hemoglobin level marks this crisis. It is common in patients with co-existent G6PD deficiency. HC is the rupturing of RBCs and the release of their contents into surround fluid (e.g. blood plasma). One cause of hemolysis is the action of hemolysins, toxins that are produced by certain pathogenic bacteria or fungi. Another cause is intense physical exercise. Hemolysins damage the RBCs. HC are acute accelerated drops in hemoglobin level. The RBCs break down at a faster rate.

Bone crisis is caused by bone marrow ischemia or infarction. These crises usually start after age 2-3 years and occur as gnawing, progressive pain, most commonly in the humerus, tibia, and femur and less commonly in the facial bones. Periarticular pain and joint effusion, often associated with a sickle cell crisis, are considered a result of ischemia and infarction of the synovium and adjacent bone and bone marrow.

Patients with acute bone pain crisis usually present with fever, leukocytosis, and warmth and tenderness around the affected joints. This process tends to affect the knees and elbows, mimicking rheumatic fever and septic arthritis.

Bone involvement is the commonest clinical manifestation of sickle cell disease both in the acute setting such as painful vaso-occlusive crises, and as a source of chronic, progressive disability such as avascular necrosis and the long-term effects of sickle cell disease on bone mineral density, growth and chronic bone and joint damage.

Orthopedic complications of sickle cell disease (SCD) include vaso-occlusive bone pain, osteonecrosis, and infections (osteomyelitis and septic arthritis).

Individuals with SCD are functionally asplenic and are at risk for infections that may be life-threatening, and other bone and joint complications can cause severe pain and immobility that significantly interfere with functioning and quality of life.

SICKLE CELL TRAIT (SCT)

What is Sickle Cell Trait?

You are born with sickle cell trait: it is inherited when only one of your parents have passed on the sickle gene, and will never develop into sickle cell disorder.

Sickle cell trait means having one gene for a condition called sickle cell disease (SCD). This in itself does not normally cause problems and sickle cell trait is not considered as a disease. It is extremely rare for it to cause problems or complications, which mainly occur under conditions of severe physical stress (explained below).

Sickle cell trait is important because your children can inherit the sickle cell gene. If BOTH parents have sickle cell trait, their children could get a double dose of the sickle cell gene, which would give them the serious condition called SCD. This is relevant if you are pregnant or wanting to start a family.

If you have the trait, the majority of red cells in the blood are normal round shaped cells. Some sickled shapes cells may be present under certain conditions. You do not have symptoms from SCT.

Sickle cell trait is found in 1 in 4 West African and 1 in 10 Afro-Caribbeans, and it is also found in people who originate from the Mediterranean, Asia and the Middle East. It is less common in white Europeans, although with the ever growing diversity of the population this will change.

Most people who have sickle cell trait are healthy. Always notify your dentist or doctor before treatment commences because anesthetics can cause problems.

There is a small chance that you may experience pain in high altitudes (generally about 10,000 feet), including long-haul flying in unpressurised planes and mountain climbing. Extreme exercise may also precipitate problems.

The trait is not an illness, but if you are planning to have children, then certain factors have to be considered. If your partner does not have SCT, then any children you have will not have SCD; but they do, your child could have the trait (50% chance)

If you and your partner both have the trait, there is a 25% chance that any child conceived may have SCD and 50% chance they will have the trait.

Sickle cell trait means that you carry a gene for a serious condition called sickle cell disease (SCD). People with sickle cell trait are well, and will usually only know about their trait if they are tested for it. Pregnant women and couples planning children may want to know whether they have sickle cell trait, because if both parents have it, their child might inherit SCD.

There is a difference with someone with Sickle Cell is SS and someone with Sickle Cell trait is AS.

However, if you want to know if your unborn child has Sickle Cell Trait (Sickle Cell Carrier) or Sickle Cell disorder, Sickle Cell Screening Tests are available.

What causes sickle cell trait and sickle cell disease (SCD)?

You inherit haemoglobin genes from both parents. One sickle cell gene gives you sickle cell trait; two sickle cell genes give you SCD.

This means that: if both parents have sickle cell trait, their children have: a 1 in 2 chance of having sickle cell trait, a 1 in 25% chance of having SCD, and a 1 in 25% chance of having no sickle genes.

If one parent has SCD and the other has sickle cell trait, their children have: a 1 in 2 chance of having sickle cell trait, and a 1 in 2 chance of having SCD.

If one parent has sickle cell trait and the other has no sickle genes, their children have: a 1 in 2 chance of having sickle cell trait, and a 1 in 2 chance of having normal haemoglobin genes.

Actually, the inheritance of SCD is slightly more complicated than that. This is because there are other haemoglobin genes which can interact with sickle cell trait. If you have one of these genes plus a sickle gene, you also get SCD (the combination behaves like two sickle cell genes). Examples of these interacting genes are HbC, beta thalassemia, Hb Lepore and HbO Arab.

How are sickle cell trait and sickle cell disease (SCD) diagnosed?

The diagnosis is made from a blood test. The blood sample is analysed to see what type of haemoglobin is present in the blood. (This is done using tests such as electrophoresis or other methods.) This can diagnose most cases of sickle cell trait and SCD.

INTRODUCTION

My name is Tola Dehinde; as someone diagnosed with the Sickle Cell genes as a baby, I know a great deal about this disorder. I know about being in and out hospital. And I also know greatly about looking after myself in order to stay out of hospital, now that I am much older.

This book is about my various experiences living with SCD and the challenges that I face and have faced as someone with Sickle Cell. My hope is to educate and inform you of tried and tested food, drinks, herbs and supplements that can make a difference in the life of someone living with Sickle Cell. I also plan to talk about living your best life while having Sickle Cell Anemia by being aware of what it is.

My aim in writing about myself in such a way, in terms of being open about how Sickle cell affects me is because I do not want anyone putting me on a pedestal. I have crises like any other person living with SCD, and in my life journey, I have decided through my writing platform to shed more light on the disease, so that we not only keep the conversation going but we can also have compassion for each other, especially if, you reading this, come across anyone with Sickle cell anemia and if you are not a SC warrior yourself.

Typically in the past, I have people come to me and talk to me about really embracing Christ because when I do, all pain will disappear. I have also had others tell me that I should not be so open. However, I want to be as real and authentic with my readers as this book is primarily for people who have Sickle cell and secondly for parents and thirdly for siblings/relatives, loved ones and friends.

Honestly, it's not been an easy road but all in all, I look back and I am thankful. I am sure if you are someone diagnosed with Sickle Cell at a young age, you don't or didn't think you will live long because you were most probably told that your life expectancy would be short; unfortunately, that has been the case for so many warriors around the world.

For those of us who are alive, I want to encourage you that life is worth living even with Sickle Cell, painful as it might be. It's not a stress-free life, as one cannot do what other people do, without falling ill sometimes. As such it is so vital to have a good care and support system in place, for those times when you need help because you are having a crisis.

Looking after yourself or having someone look after you or care for you is so important in the life of someone with Sickle Cell. Mothers and fathers who care for their child or children from the moment they were diagnosed with Sickle Cell do an incredibly decent work.

I remember my mum would 'force' me to eat what is 'good for me'; the fact that my mum was a nurse also helped. Fast forward to now, five decades plus down the line, I have become a fussy and picky eater, thanks mum!

I am all for eating well and eating good food that is nutritious and will help me stay out of hospital. And also I am all for eating food that will help the sickle shaped blood cells in my body not clot, so that if I am in pain at home, it is only a mini crisis. Truthfully, sometimes despite my best efforts, I still fall ill and do end up in hospital. As they say, c'est la vie – that's life.

If you suffers from Sickle Cell, then you know how to look after yourself:

Keep warm, don't over stretch yourself, don't get too excited, eat well and drink plenty of fluid, preferably water, in order to keep your blood cells moving and not clot.

Most importantly, try and walk away from stress, warriors cannot handle too much stress and also if you are feeling tired, give yourself the rest that your body needs.

PART 1: SICKLE CELL AND MY PERSONAL EXPERIENCE

Here I was in the middle of summer and I felt pains in my left thigh and before I knew what was going on, I was dragging that leg painfully across my apartment. I knew, this was a full blown crisis coming up. I sent texts to a few close friends and family members, to let them know what was going on. After two days of taking Morphine, Codeine and all other painkillers that I could lay my hands on, this pain was getting progressively worse, I knew I had to go into hospital.

One of my friends who lives abroad called me and I told her that I needed to go to hospital and she quickly called her daughter to come over to mine and we were able to call an ambulance. I was taken to the hospital I attend, where I was admitted to the ward. I was in hospital for four days.

I try to go for my Haemotology out-patients quarterly clinic check-up and rarely get admitted into hospital for a full blown crisis. The hospital has improved and keeps on improving its heamotology department. While admitted, I found out they now have a Haemotology pain clinic, opened seven days a week from 8 am till 8 pm. I thought, this is great for those who work. How I wish this was available when I was still in full-time employment.

Sickle Cell and the Day Pain Clinic

Six months or so later, I was sick again and called the pain clinic, as that is the protocol. When you call, they ask for your details and then wait for you to turn up. You are not allowed to just turn up without phoning first. So, when I got there, they knew I was not in a state for any long talk, I just wanted this crazy pain to leave my body. I gave them my hospital number and within 10 minutes, I am being given my first Morphine injection and within another hour I was given another injection and then about two hours later, I was given a third and last Morphine injection for the day. The idea is to act fast and furiously by bombarding the pain with shots of morphine.

After the third Morphine shot, I was totally drugged up and the pain had eased off slightly. I was kept under observation for an hours or so after. A friend later came to pick me up at the hospital and brought me home. I got home and went straight to bed. The next morning, I called the pain clinic again and informed them that I will be there later that morning, as the pain had not gone. I got there and they followed the previous day's procedure. The thing is, if I had gone for three day consecutively, they would have admitted me into hospital. So, on the third day, I rested at home and went back on the fourth day, knowing that I could look after myself at home, after going to the pain clinic three times that week. To me, the pain clinic is a life-saver.

During my three days of going back and forth at the haemotology pain clinic, I saw people coming and going and I could tell some people were coming from work and it was great to see this going on.

Sickle Cell is draining on one's pocket. Going to the hospital three times that week, having to take a taxi back home cost money. Eating healthy meals in order to look after yourself cost money. Taking supplements also cost money.

When I was working full-time, there was only the option of admission into hospital when I was sick. Working for a big corporate media organization meant being by-passed on promotion because of being off sick a lot from work.

The management of Sickle Cell cannot stay the same and medical doctors all over the world are really trying to find a cure and also help us with Sickle Cell manage the pains better. I found the fact that doctors and nurses were willing to give me Morphine, without my shouting the ward or A&E down, very uplifting.

Back in the day, when I used to be sick a lot, some twenty years ago, doctors were reluctant to prescribe Morphine to people with Sickle Cell, because of fear of dependency. I heard it said that people with Sickle Cell become addicted to Morphine, which has the street name for Heroine. All I know is that when I am in pain, I need Morphine!

Sickle Cell and my Childhood

Today, I would like to talk about how tough it can be living with Sickle Cell. The exasperating thing about Sickle Cell is how it creeps up on one unexpectedly. Now that I am mature, I know the tell-tale signs and quickly deal with them.

But when I was a child, I didn't know the tell-tale signs and as such, I remember falling ill just before my older siblings birthday parties or before an important event was about to take place or after something important had taken place in the family. My childhood was characterized with being sick often enough but I had love and everyone knew to look after me in the house.

The hard part of living with Sickle Cell is that one minute all is okay and the next minute, I have to be carried to the bathroom or toilet or need someone to get something for me. It is degrading and embarrassing, being grown up and yet being so helpless because of pain. The pain could start from any part of my body, it could start with my hand, shoulder, knee, back, chest etc… and before I know it the pain has spread all my body and I cannot move or do anything for myself. What kind of sickness is this? A sickness that totally incapacitates the sufferer; how can this be?

When I have a full blown crisis, everyone would look at me with pity in their eyes because there is nothing that they can do to take the pain away. It is brutal, to have a loved one, sister, brother, child, wife, husband, cousin who has Sickle Cell, and there is nothing you can do to help when he or she is sick.

And that is why we call ourselves warriors. The pain is indescribable, unapologetic and brutal. I always think of it as a hurricane.

I remember when I was a child and in my teens, when I became ill with a full blown crisis, what I wanted the most was for someone to put something heavy on my back. I needed some really heavy weight on my back and would hope and pray that the weight will suppress the pain. Of course my loved ones did not want to put a BIG box or suitcase on the back of someone who is ill, sick, frail, weak and a light weight. However I needed this pain subdued and quashed because, if either of these two things didn't happen, I would die of the pain infiltrating my body. Of course I did not die but that was how I felt at the height of the pain, when much younger.

I remember going to a party a long time ago, all well dressed and dancing to the beat of the music and before I knew what was going on, here I was 'displaying' at someone's party. What I mean is having a full blown crisis and being unable to sit still. I look back and can only laugh at my adventures with Sickle Cell.

This sickness is so unbelievably crippling and that is the part of Sickle Cell that I find hard to comprehend. One minute, you are playing as a child with your friends and the next minute, BAM, you are down health wise.

Or as an adult, one minute I am working hard at work and overnight, the crisis hits me and I am unable to go to work the following day. How do I explain it to your boss? Someone who knows nothing about Sickle Cell and could be thinking that I am lying that I am truly sick. Afterall, if you have a cold or a cough, it does not start suddenly.

Sickle Cell is much more than a cold or cough though. Eventually, I always get better, go back to work and work even harder because I am trying to overcompensate for being sick, when having Sickle Cell is my reality.

Sometimes, unfortunately, a lot of things that I would want to do, I cannot do. Painful as Sickle Cell is, I want to encourage anyone who knows someone who has Sickle Cell to please cut them some slack.

A lot of people have died from the disease, so if you know someone who is alive and keeping it together, working, striving, studying, hopeful, not giving up, such a person deserves more of your encouragement and less of your criticism because you don't know if the person was in pain all through the night and still showed up in the morning, weak and tired but showed up.

Sickle Cell and Christmas 2016

Here I was, getting ready for Christmas 2016 and I went last minute shopping with my cousin two days before Xmas, in the morning. Got back home and as I was removing my outdoor clothes, I could feel some pain here and there. Didn't think much of it, but took some pain killers, just to be on the safe side and had a very hot shower, in the hope that whatever it was, would disappear as suddenly as it came.

I had a bad night and spent the day Christmas eve, all curled up in pain and taking strong painkillers. Come Xmas day, it was a Sunday and off I made my way to church, even though, I was terribly unwell. After church, I make my way over to see someone who was ill. After it was off for a lovely Xmas lunch at my cousin's. Again, I was pretending to be well, when in actual fact, I should have stayed home. Sickle Cell wasn't going to make me stay home on Xmas day I kept telling myself. I will and most conquer this sickness and show it who is boss were my thoughts.

Unfortunately though, I had to leave 'the Xmas party' early because as the day wore on, I was in a very bad way. For starters, all the layers that I had on, felt so uncomfortable, my body was telling me to get these clothes off.

I got home, took the clothes off right away, had another very hot shower, trying desperately to help those blood cells that are clotted, unclog themselves. I took more Morphine tablets and laid myself down in pain. I took tablets from then till after Boxing Day. I had to admit defeat and made my way to the pain clinic on the 27th of December.

And that is how the festive season passed me by. All the things I wanted to do at the end of the year, I had to be put on hold, as I recovered. And that was how instead of being in church for the watch night service, I was home watching a watch night service on the television. How nice!

Here I am, it's a new year and I am getting better day by day and recovering, as I am also getting stronger as each day passes by. I am sleeping a lot in order to get all the Morphine taken out of my system.

I feel very positive about 2017, I just do. So this year, I have decided to make sure that I take on exercise and by that I mean walking. I read somewhere, that walking is the best form of exercise. I do not do any such thing as power walking but I walk at my leisure. Especially now as I am trying to get my strength back, it is important that I go out, get some fresh air and energize my organs. I walk for about 30 minutes to an hour, it all depends on my physical capability on the day.

Sickle Cell and my New Year Resolution

On a personal note, this year is going to be about looking after every area of my life. I am not talking about just eating well. I keep repeating this, Sickle Cell does not like stress, and so if you are eating well, exercising but you are not trying to get rid of stress in your life, then you will fall ill and that was what happened to me.

This year, I am going to focus on the things that really matter: life, health, positive relationships and work. In the middle of it all, if my body tells me it needs a break or a rest, I intend to stop what I am doing and give it the rest it deserves.

If I find that I am stressed about a matter, I will walk away from it. I cannot afford to be sick in the middle of important events in my life. No, this year, I will not be giving stress the time nor day. I need to get back into focus, I can't blame Sickle Cell for me taking my eyes off, looking after myself; so my message to you adults who understand where I am coming from is, let's be progressive with Sickle Cell and no blame game.

Sickle Cell and my
First Blood Transfusion

There is something about sickle cell and it is about the individual nature of the disease. People ask me questions about blood transfusion and sickle cell. If you are fortunate to have lived long, (I mean if you are over forty), you will most definitely have stories to tell about sickle cell showing you up at one time or the other of your life.

Let me tell you the story of my first blood transfusion a very long time ago; I must have been in my mid-twenties. A lot of people with sickle cell can go through life without having blood transfusion. However, from time to time a blood transfusion may be required, either because the anemia has become worse or to lower the level of sickle haemoglobin in the blood or because your packed cell volume (PCV) is low.

People with Sickle Cell Disease have sickle haemoglobin (HbSS) which can make red blood cells rigid and sickle-shaped so they cannot bend and flex easily through normal red blood cells. This can lead to small blood vessels getting blocked that in turn can lead to severe painful crisis. This can also cause damage to organs such as the liver, kidney, lungs, heart, brain and spleen.

So back to my story, here I was on this fateful day, admitted into hospital with a crisis. The doctor finally came to see me after they have done all the tests they needed to do and he told me that I would need a blood transfusion.

I heard the words 'blood transfusion' and started crying and going hysterical. All my life, my mother had raised me and made sure that I was well looked after; she had taken care of me at home, being that she was a nurse. I had never had to have a blood transfusion till this particular time.

So, here I was in a foreign land, a long way away from home and I'm being told, I needed blood transfusion. My goodness! I was crying, hyperventilating and forgot about the Sickle Cell pain, as I equated, in my mind blood transfusion with HIV! How ignorant of me. I thought to myself, I am going to die with this transfusion. The unfortunate thing at the time was I was all alone, I had no one with me to reassure me, ask questions on my behalf and here I was being given this bombshell. When in pain, you forget to ask the questions that you need answers to. What shall I do? Should I say yes to this thing or say no for religious reasons? I struggled in my mind with what to do for ages.

Initially, the doctor thought I was crying because of the pain and he kept trying to reassure me down and was telling me that it was the best they could do for me, because my blood level was very low. He continued, that as they try to control the pain, it was also necessary for me to be given top up blood. I eventually voiced my concern to the doctor who did his best to alleviate my fears.

I ultimately said yes because they were worried about me. As I was given the transfusion, I kept looking at the blood bag and the drip like it was a death trap. I didn't expect to live, can you imagine how ill-informed I was back then? Of course, I did not die then and I am still very much alive decades later, having had blood transfusion a few more times since then.

We will look into the difference between a blood transfusion and blood exchange later on in this book, as I have had both.

Knowledge they say is power and so if you suffer from sickle cell and need transfusion or you are looking after a loved one who has been recommended for a blood transfusion, get medical advice and help yourself or your loved one.

And if you are reading this and do not have Sickle cell, then perhaps you could also do some research on giving blood.

Sickle Cell and Vision Loss

Some years ago, I had a sickle cell crisis and had to be admitted into hospital. I was there for a week. On the day that I was being discharged, I noticed that I had gone blind in my left eye. Strange I thought, as this had never happened to me before. Since the incident, I found out that it does happen to people living with sickle cell and sadly it is one of the complications of SCD.

I waited for a couple of weeks to see if I would regain my sight but nothing happened. As far as I know, it did not get worse, neither did it get better, I still could not see with my left eye. I was then advised to go and see an ophthalmologist. I was abroad at the time and did not feel comfortable going to see someone who did not know my history. I decided to come back to London.

Immediately, I settled down, I went to the haematology outpatient department of the hospital that I normally attend and explained to my doctor what had happened. I was referred straightaway to the specialist eye hospital. I went, they did a scan of my eye and explained that I had 'vitreous haemorrhage'; the name alone was scary. I had what? I kept thinking was there no end to the complications of Sickle Cell?! How can I have a crisis and then end up losing my vision?

I was told that there was no medical treatment, except surgery. I was informed that with time, the blood from my retina would clear by itself and my vision will be restored but it would several months. I was given appointments every six weeks or so and I attended them all.

The consultant then said that they could operate on my eye, in order to remove the blood from my retina, if I wished, however, I was also told that once they started 'touching' my eye, then all kinds of complications could start occurring with the eye.

By then though, I had started to see little by little and so I declined surgery. I then took the executive decision to weather this 'new' storm; I will see again; my left eye will function normally again; I kept saying and repeating to myself. Eventually, as months went by, I started seeing more and more. It was like a flower bud opening up. It took a long time, well over six months and it was a horrible experience.

At the time, if you looked at my left eye, it looked normal, but I could only see bloodshot and nothing else. The experience was extremely distressing and traumatic. I would be out and about, and someone would just go by and I had no idea that the person was passing by, I felt so vulnerable when I was out in public and hardly went out. I stayed home a lot during that time.

Those months were tough, especially for someone who had no vision problems for over four decades. I had an appreciation of what blind people go through. Here I am today, thankful that I am seeing perfectly well once again.

One thing that I have realised with Sickle Cell is that you do have to have loved ones' close by and around you, always, for such a time as when you need help and support. I have friends who will do some shopping for me when I am sick. My pantry is always full, because I always think of times when I am sick and I cannot go food shopping.

What Then Is Vitreous Haemorrhage?

"Blood cells that change shape, or "sickle," can get trapped in blood vessels, blocking the blood flow. When this blockage occurs in the small blood vessels in the inner lining (retina) of the eyes, it can cause vision problems. This most often occurs in people who have hemoglobin SC disease, a type of sickle cell disease. In the worst cases, the retina may come loose, leading to permanent blindness. This may happen suddenly, without any warning."

Vitreous haemorrhage is bleeding or occurs when blood leaks into the vitreous humour inside the eye. The blood most commonly comes from blood vessels at the back of the eye. This substance is the vitreous humour. It helps the eye keep its shape and is normally clear, allowing light from outside the eye to pass through it to reach the retina.

Vitreous haemorrhage varies in degree from mild, with 'floaters' and haziness in the vision, to complete loss of vision. It is painless and it comes on quite quickly. Usually only one eye is affected. Whilst it is very alarming, once the bleeding has been treated, many cases resolve and vision is restored to where it was before. In order for us to see clearly, the vitreous humour needs to be clear. If the vitreous humour is clouded or filled with blood, vision will be impaired. This varies from a few 'floaters' and cloudiness of the vision through to the vision going completely dark (sometimes with a reddish tinge).

Sickle Cell and the Shadow of Death

So here I was at the end of July of this particular year, I had gone away for the weekend and had a really fabulous time. I got back home early evening on the Sunday and within 30 minutes, I was having chest pain (which I have never had), ribs pain and back pain. No symptoms, no warning, nothing. All at once and the pain was so overwhelming that I was finding it difficult to breath and could barely speak, as every time I spoke, the pain that was already 10/10 felt as if it was 20/10; completely inexpressible, how does one describe a pain that makes an adult cry?

I quickly took painkillers but the pains did not subside. I thought I can't sleep in my house tonight, I have to call an ambulance and let them come and get me. But yours truly persevered in pain all night, as deep down, I did not want to get admitted into hospital. To top it all, I had no one around. This wasn't good.

As the dawn set in on Monday, I was happy to see the daylight break through the darkness of the night. It had been a sleepless and long night of pain and waiting. I quickly called the Haemotology day pain clinic. I have to call the clinic before I make my way there and go through some checks with the nurse over the phone.

When I got there they had already prepared the intravenous morphine injection that they were going to give me. Usually, I try as much as possible to not go to the pain clinic unless absolutely necessary. Typically, when I present myself at the pain clinic, I would have been at home, in pain, for some days.

Prior to this particular admission, I had seen my consultant during my outpatients' appointment a month earlier. I mentioned to him, that by the time I make my way to the day clinic, I would have been in pain, at home for a few days. I then asked if he could increase the amount of morphine that I am given, when I come to the pain clinic. I usually use 10mgs at home and when I come to the hospital, I told him I wanted a higher dose and he agreed and wrote in my hospital file that I could be given up 20 mgs. 'Up to' being the operative words in this situation.

Back to my story, bearing in mind that I had been self-medicating at home to no avail, I arrived at the pain clinic in agony and holding back my tears because of the pain. I am once again impressed by their ability to inject the first dose of morphine within 15 minutes of my getting there. The nurse decided to give me 20 mgs. Days like this, I am not really with it and I am sure you can understand why.

After an hour had passed by, she proceeded to give me the 2nd morphine injection, again 20 mgs. I am still in pain and I am quietly praying that this next injection will turn things around, for the better, for me. Each time after I am given the injections, I am checked to make sure my blood pressure, heart beat etc... are all working and in order.

Now, after about two and a half hours, this same nurse comes to administer the third and last injection and once again, she gives me 20 mgs. This meant, that in such a short period of time, less than five hours, my body had been pumped with 60 mgs of morphine. The dose was too much for me and as a nurse she should have known better. Due to the fact that I was in a lot of pain, I did not ask questions as I would normally do.

By then, I was throwing up profusely, as if my guts wanted to come out of me; don't forget that I had not eaten anything since the day before. I was sweating profusely as well and it was general pain and discomfort all over my body. I was in an out of slumber, drugged up and not really paying attention to anything. Shortly after this third and last injection for the day, something happened and I was unaware of it.

The Morphine was an overdose and I 'died' in medical terms, on two separate occasions. What I became aware of was opening my eyes to see doctors and nurses surrounding the bed I was on. I saw the doctors and nurses telling me what had happened.

I looked at them, puzzled, wondering what was going on. Then one of the doctors told me that I had I reacted to the morphine given to me and had been declared clinically dead. This was because they had been calling my name for a few minutes apparently, this doctor said and I had not responded. Well, I did not hear anyone calling my name or putting their hands on me.

Too much morphine had been administered into me and within a short period of time and hence the overdose. I thought, 'excuse me, you guys overdosed me.' I was fuming but I was too weak to talk, argue, fight my corner, assert myself with these people. They were mindful to not put the blame on themselves but to tell me that I reacted to morphine. I of course understand that this had not been intentional but accidental negligence.

They wanted to take me straight up to the HDU (high dependency unit); I was like dependency what? No, I am not going there.

I walked here this morning and will be walking out this afternoon, to go home, get some rest and maybe come over tomorrow, if this mind-blowing pain is still there, I said.

They argued with me but I was adamant and then they said ok but I need to be observed and they kept me in the pain clinic till just before they closed at eight pm. Usually, once I have had the three injections, I come back home in the afternoon to rest and sleep the morphine off.

After they all left my bedside, insisting that I was not going to spend the night in hospital, to be monitored, the realization of what had happened hit me. My goodness! I could have died, just like that and that would have been it. I just started crying silently as I thanked God.

The following day, I stayed away because to be frank with you, having had that near death experience with no one around, I was freaked out and just thought 'bear the pain at home Tola'. Of course the pain was still very much there and so went back on Wednesday, where I had a nurse who decided to be overly careful and give me 10mg, 12.5mg and 10mg again, which did not suppress the pain one bit.

But again, I was too weak to be arguing and the Monday experience was in the nurse's mind and mine and so I just left it because I knew where she was coming from; better safe than sorry was her approach.

I stayed indoors on Thursday and went to the pain clinic again on Friday. All the nurses had heard about the patient who 'overdosed' on Morphine and they were now being very careful. The nurse on Friday gave me 15mg three times and that seem to work for me. By the end of that day, I knew I could recover and get well at home.

I deliberated in my mind, why that particular nurse could not think things through? Why did she not go and consult with a Haemotology doctor before she gave me the second and third morphine injection, as she would have noticed that my frame is rather small? My doctor had put in my notes/folder, up to 20 mg, meaning anything from 10 – 20 mgs. Do I have to become a nurse now, in order to make sure Sickle cell patients get good enough care? Though she started with 20 mgs, she could have reduced it to 10 mgs for the remaining two injections, could she not? I had lots of questions in my mind, but there was no one to answer them because I did not have the strength to demand answers on what happened.

I am writing about this particular experience because I want to implore you reading, if you know someone with SS who has a hospital appointment; if you are close enough to that person, and can volunteer the time, then try and go to hospital with the patient as Sickle cell crises can be debilitating.

And if you are a Sickle cell patient, (old enough to go to hospital on your own), try and see if you have someone who can accompany you to the hospital, (this is not always possible, I know, as crisis can occur, without warning). Try not go on your own, where you sometimes have to make serious decisions when you are most vulnerable and sick.

The fact that I am sick and have to go to hospital, does not mean that everyone around me have to stop living their lives and pander to my needs. I understand that it not possible. If you have Sickle cell, hospital is not a strange place to you; you thereby think that it is safe to go on your own, right, but not so. The purpose of this write-up is to tell you all to be mindful when going into hospital and as per usual, I am still in the land of the living and fighting on.

Sickle Cell and a Day in my Life

As you may know or not, a lot of people who suffer from Sickle cell go through pains on a constant basis and yet keep on with their business and hence their getting the nickname 'warrior'. A lot of people go through discomforts of some sort and yet, will go to work or any other business that they have going on because they do not want to disappoint anyone, and they continue with their lives despite the odds and the pains they are going through.

I had been feeling unwell for some weeks now and I know the telltale signs if it's going to lead to a crisis and I try to take care of it as quickly as I can. Regarding this situation, I would say that I was feeling extra weak, tired, lethargic and more pronounced pain in all my joints but kept about my business. It had actually gotten to the point where I was medicating at home on morphine and codeine; but I would still go to work and come back home and crash at home after a day's work. Normally, I try to nip it in the bud pretty quickly, but this time, I was popping pills and the pains were not getting any better but I was preoccupied with life and I didn't pay much attention to it as I normally would have.

Then one night, as I was unable to sleep (nothing new), I heard a voice ask me if I was going to let myself die this way? As you can imagine, I was startled about what I heard and decided that night, that as soon as it was daybreak, I would start getting ready, so that by 8 am, I would call the day pain clinic and take it from there. Well that is the life of someone with SCD; always erratic and totally unpredictable at best.

I sent a text to a good friend in the early hours of the morning asking if she could drop me at the hospital in a few hours' time. My friend replied and said no problems and I started getting myself ready. She arrived later on and off we went, getting to the hospital by 8.20 am. I was early, there was no nurse about and so, sat waiting in the reception area, as I had called them to inform them I would be coming over.

Eventually, all nurses started trickling in and I finally got attended to. As they take my blood, I told them to not give me any morphine shot without first given me an anti-sickness injection. The nurse did and said she will have to wait for it to kick in before she gives me the morphine injection; I was happy with that. In the meantime, she was putting a cannula in my arm as she was looking for a vein.

Once she found it, I was given some IV paracetamol and a shot of morphine. When the blood result came back, by this time, I had been given the first shot of morphine, I am told that my blood and iron levels were all very low.

I am like wow! Ok, so how had I been coping and pushing myself for such a while? As a result, the consultant hematologist and other doctors come to me. The consultant told me that he would like to keep me in and I told him no. On that first day, they were able to give me top-up iron IV. They wanted me in the next day, so I could be given about two pints of blood. By the end of the first day, I had been given so many injections, blood had been taken for various tests and all these took several attempts because my veins have always been difficult to find. I went home stressed out, weak, bruised and tired and still in pain.

I had made sure to ask, as I was being given morphine injections, I was also given anti-sickness injections; the nurse told me the anti-sickness injection last for 6-8 hours.

So, on my way home, I was so sure about not throwing up. I was wrong, just as I was getting home, I could feel something coming up. I had put an extra plastic bag in my main bag and just put it around my mouth and quickly rushed indoors, as I did not want to start throwing up in public.

I therefore got home and as I was being fussed over, I had to rush past the open front door, and made my way to the bathroom because I had stuff in my mouth.

I went back to the pain clinic on the second day and again got there by about 8.30 am. I was still in pain and they did what they normally do in order to relieve the pain that I was going through. By then, they had taken more blood samples. Not too long after, they came back worried (they being the medical team) because my blood level had further gone down, compared to the previous day. I knew in my heart that nothing was going to happen to me as this too shall pass. I was told I would have to be given some blood.

Once the pain had subsided, then it was time to send off for a cross-match. This is a procedure where before a blood transfusion takes place, a test is done, in order to determine if the donor's blood is compatible with the blood of an intended recipient. After this process, then the blood transfusion started. This took a while and as the blood transfusion was taking place, they made sure that they were constantly checking my oxygen and blood pressure levels in order to ascertain that all was ok.

After spending about eight hours in hospital, the one pint of transfusion was complete and I was allowed to leave and go home. I got home tired, went to bed and slept off.

The same process was followed on the third day and after that, I knew that all what I needed to do was recover at home and look after myself as well as I could.

By that, I mean, eating well because truth be told, I had been given so many pain relieving injections over the three days and tablets that I was just sick and tired of anything to do with medication and wanted to eat myself to recovery. But of course, eating is not always appealing when one is not well and one hasn't got an appetite but eat I must.

I believe in healthy eating and the reason why I talk a lot about food is not because I particularly love food but because I realise that if I want to live a relatively healthy life, in spite of Sickle cell, then I needed to be mindful of what I eat.

Also, perhaps because of the strong opioids that I take, I tend to be bloated, constipated or I throw up quite a lot; this therefore means, I need to understand more about food and my gut.

Sickle Cell and my Faith

Even though I have lived with Sickle Cell for over five decades, it is a disease that I know so well and yet sometimes, it is totally unfathomable to me, in terms of the pain and the precariousness of Sickle Cell disorder.

When I was growing up, it was about Tola, you can't do this or Tola you can't do that and if I disobeyed and played rough as a child with other kids, I would feel the brunt of what I did, that I should not have done at night when I had a crisis. And you know the African mother will not nurse you without telling you 'did I not warn you?' Tact is the last thing to expect from an African mother even in the midst of their child crying out in pain. Now, to the adult human mind, that makes sense, I should not have done something strenuous but I was a child and wanted to play with my friends.

But how can I explain that I am well one minute, watching TV, texting or talking to a friend and I go into my kitchen to get something and as I enter the kitchen, I feel a sharp pain that was not there when I walked from the living room. Or I'm downstairs and walk up the stairs to my bedroom and tales of the unexpected happen, sharp pain as I sit on the bed.

Or I wake up in the morning, and get ready for work, make my way out and as I walk to my car parked on the street, a short distance from home and as I open the car door and sit in the car, about to turn the ignition on and guess what, that sharp pain emerges.

Now that is the thing about Sickle Cell that drives me nuts. How can one have a good quality of life when one does not know from one minute to the next, whether one is going to be alright or not? And subconsciously as a result, I don't and can't make long term plans. I really don't book anything months in advance but a few weeks before the event itself, especially if I have to pay.

I have over the years been sick, at home, unable to go to work but will get up in the evening, get dressed to go to church and teach Bible study; finish my assignment at church and gently make my way back home and crawl back into bed. What I have noticed is that people with Sickle Cell either love God or have this love/hate relationship with God.

As for me, I choose to serve God in the midst of this world that makes no sense and in the middle of the physical pain that I go through daily. I can't hate God because He is all I have supernaturally speaking. He is the One who has kept me alive, when I was sick as a child and everyone around me thought, I would die. He is the One who watched over me and made it possible for me to work for decades despite Sickle Cell and its challenges. He is the One who is with me, when I am in a hospital bed or on my bed at home languishing in pain.

Before I was, God existed and He knows me and see me and communes with me. I have decided to praise Him through my circumstance, ill or well.

As you can tell, I have a strong faith and sometimes, that inner critical voice would tell me to curse God and die. Or it would ask me why am I serving a God who says He heals and yet I am not healed because believe me when I tell you I have prayed and other people have prayed too.

I have been to prayer mountains, I have been for deliverances, I have had hands laid on me, drank Holy water and anointing oil. You name it, church wise, I have done it and still Sickle Cell keeps rearing its ugly head in my physical body.

The Bible tells me that God is a Spirit and those who worship Him, must do so in spirit and in truth and that is my testimony, worshipping Him in spirit and in truth and to keep being a light that shines in the Lord.

Jesus in his days did not heal everybody; some people got their healing and some didn't. Does that mean, that because Jesus did not heal everyone, he is not God? Of course He is. As we know, rain falls on the just and the unjust.

For me, it's about holding on to God as my Anchor. Being sick after having prayed is nothing to do with having less faith but more to do with God who tells me that His grace is sufficient for me during the good and bad times.

God loves us all the same irrespective of what our struggles are in life and so, let's be sensitive to those who are sick and stop the Bible bashing by saying to someone he/she has no faith because they are not well. Some will die young and some old, some will die at middle age and some within a few hours on this earth; that is life. But more than anything, if you know someone who has Sickle Cell, do pick up the phone from time to time and ask after their wellbeing. The phone call, the encouraging word, the offer to assist, the love offering, the cooking, cleaning, whatever you can do for someone who is unwell, goes a long way.

Sickle Cell and my Mother

It has taken me a lot to get my mother to pen down my birth and all. However, after much persuasion and series of 'I can'ts', she finally agreed. Enjoy her personal account of having a child with Sickle Cell: I got married to my late husband, ambassador Dehinde in England. We have four children and Tola is the third child.

We never knew that my husband and I were Sickle Cell carriers, until we had Tola. When she was about one year's old, I noticed her hands and feet would swell on and off (hand-foot syndrome) and they would be tender to touch. Being a trained nurse, I told my husband that it is likely Tola has Sickle Cell disease.

I went to our doctor, who then referred us to the hospital that specialises in children sicknesses, to this day (Great Ormond Street hospital – GOSH). There, they did a genotype test and we were told that she has HbSS. We were also tested and we both found out we had the SC trait. Subsequently, I started taking her to the hospital, the out patients department for her appointments.

We eventually came back to Lagos and I brought her case notes with me. I started taking her to see the late Dr Olukoye Ransome-Kuti (a pediatrician) at the Lagos University Teaching hospital (LUTH), where I had previously worked. In due course, I had to give up the nursing profession, because of the unpredictable nature of Sickle Cell crisis in Tola's life.

All the time, she was having crisis on and off, I looked after her and nursed her at home. This was with the help of my late mother, my siblings, other relations and friends who were always there for us, to lend helping hands anytime she had these attacks of gruesome and excruciating pains.

When she was much younger, anytime she had these Sickle Cell crisis, the whole family would be destabilised. This meant, that when we wanted to do anything in the family, with her condition, it was only God who saw us through because Tola would fall sick either before or right after the event. When she had a crisis, Tola would cry and this meant sleepless nights for her and others in the house. She would ask us to sit on her back, hold her legs, hands or rub her with some analgesic ointment to no avail, as she did not get any relief. These crises would sometimes come without warning and leave suddenly; the duration would always vary. This affected Tola's schooling as her attendance was not 100%. As soon as she got better, she would go about her business as a child (school and playing), just as if nothing had happened but leaving the rest of us tired and weak.

I was always quite apprehensive when we had something coming up in the family because of Tola. As we did not know if she would be able to withstand the family function, or if she would be ill. As she grew up, the crises were not as frequent and as such, she was able to pay her last respect during my mother's and her dad's funerals without being sick.

I was strict with her diet when she was growing up and she jokes now, that she is a fussy eater because of all the things that I made sure her eat when she was living under our roof.

When Tola was young, I made sure I fed her with a balanced diet, filled with protein like liver, beans, meat and chicken. I also made sure the food were rich in calcium for her bones and teeth (milk and eggs). I gave her carbohydrate rich food, like yam, potatoes, sweet corn, yam flour (iyan), cassava flour (elubo), rice, all manner of green vegetables, namely: tete, ewuro, ewedu, soko and okra. I also made sure she ate plenty of fruits in season.

I would have to force her to take her tablets when she was young as she hated taking medicines. With what she went through, Tola was frequently sick but she managed to finish her primary and secondary education. She later travelled out of the country where she went to university, through God's mercy and grace.

I am eternally grateful to God for sparing her life till today and for making her a living testimony. I am proud of her as a mother. I encourage all children with Sickle Cell and their parents all over the world to not lose hope.

Sickle Cell and Flying

Here I was one day recently, tens of thousands of feet up in the air (I was travelling by plane). When I bid my family farewell at the airport of departure, I was well and doing ok, health wise. Suddenly, about four hours to landing, I was sleeping and felt pain in my feet. I'm a light sleeper; maybe it's because of having Sickle Cell crises through the years starting at night. Nonetheless, I know my body well enough to realize that something negative was about to happen and I was miles away from dry land. I then thought, it's nothing T, go back to sleep.

I could not go back to sleep because the pain was intense and was now moving up my body and before I knew it, all my body was in severe agony. I sighed and wondered what should I do? Then I remembered that I had opiate tablets in my bag. I quickly looked for them, everyone around me was asleep because it was in the middle of the night. I could not get up, the throbbing pain was that much. So, I hoped that an air hostess would walk by.

After what seems like a lifetime (it was actually minutes), one walked by and I stopped her. I told her I was unwell and needed some water and some biscuits. I am one of those who cannot swallow tablets without some food. Anyway, she brought what I had requested and I quickly took the anti-sickness tablet and the opiate tablet, one after the other.

I then waited for the tablet to work its magic and for the pain to go from a ten to at least a five. As I was waiting, I was also hoping that my body would not reject this opiate. As it was, I didn't feel nauseous and for that I was grateful.

After a short period of time, I could feel the intense pain easing off. Thank goodness for that. I could no longer sleep as this episode had woken me up.

Finally the plane landed and I go off the plane. By then, I had taken another set of lesser pain-killers as I did not want to be spaced out when landing and behaving funny at the airport.

I got someone to help me pick my suitcases and lift them onto the trolley. I then called a taxi and eventually got to my destination. The driver was kind enough to carry my suitcases right to my front door for me. Those two random acts of not picking my suitcases up at the airport and also of not carrying them myself to the front door, were acts of kindness that meant either going to hospital or not. Once indoors, I took care of myself as I always do, took a very hot shower as this helps me to no end and then ate and took more opiate. And the rest as they say is history.

Now as we landed, I sent a text to my support group who needed to know that I had landed but unwell. This brings me to the issue of who are your support group, if you have sickle cell? You don't need to have a lot of people but enough who can be there for you, if need be.

I mean in terms of helping you buy your tablets from the chemist, go shopping or bring you some food or help you out financially (if that is what you need) because having a long-term illness does not come cheap, in terms of buying tablets, eating good food or going to the chemist or taking a taxi to the hospital when sick. Or someone who can stand in the gap for you spiritually. I encourage young adults to have a support group of three to four people who can be of assistance in their time of need.

If you are reading this and you don't have this, please look into having a support group. To have to go out and buy tablets for yourself when you are in pain is tough and I am speaking as someone who knows.

While I am on this crusade for every warrior to have a support group, could I also ask that if you are reading this and know someone who has sickle cell or you know a parent who has a child/ren with sickle cell, do extend a helping hand.

Ask them what help they need, don't guess. Everyone's needs are different and so help will also differ. But more than anything, do ask how someone with sickle cell is doing from time to time because you don't know, they might just be sick. Take my case for example, I boarded the plane in good form and came off it sick.

Sickle Cell and Tales of the Unexpected

It is a fact that Sickle Cell is no respecter of person, time or place; this means a painful Sickle Cell episode can occur anywhere and at any time. Over the years, I have been careless and care free to the point whereby I have had crises that I should not have had, if only I had looked after myself better. Thank goodness for God's grace over me.

But now, being older and wiser, I realise I cannot be careless with my body or lifestyle and I have a duty to take care of myself, as much as I can. Over the years, I have had one incident after another; to the point where I don't sleep out any longer. The reason is because I could be somewhere and have a crisis, in someone else's home, something I detest.

One of such days, here I was, far away from home and I was staying with one of my numerous older sisters. Nowadays, I tell myself, if I am sick, let it be in the comfort of my home and not me humiliating myself in someone else's home; actually it's Sickle Cell shaming itself.

Anyway, back to my story, I was staying with my cousin and all of a sudden, this silly thing raised its ugly head. Sometimes, before I know what is going on, my body is on fire within minutes. Or I could be thinking ok, Tola brace yourself, still trying to catch my breath and wonder what I need to do in order to nip this pain in the bud. But if the pain shoots up from one to ten, within the twinkle of an eye, days like that, I know this crisis has arrived with a vengeance.

I know the drill and know in my heart that this is not unto death, even though the pain is so much that talking is a no no and the only thing I can do is cry out in pain with the inability to not stay still. So, one minute I am on the bed, the next minute, on the floor, the next minute sitting in the bathroom floor, on the toilet seat and basically trying to find awkward positions that I think might somehow ease the pain in my body. If you have had a Sickle Cell crisis, you most probably understand what I am talking about.

The concern though is when I have people around me. I feel for whoever is with me when sick at home. I am not talking of being in hospital because there I would be given injections to curb the pain. But at home, sometimes, the pain relieving tablets do not work. In the midst of my pain, I am being a contortionist because of the mind blowing throbbing pain wreaking havoc through my body.

My people know me to be fiercely independent and so they don't know this Tola who is crying, screaming in pain and can't sit still. They don't understand it and I can imagine that it must be really hard to watch a loved one going through such torture. My distress rubs off on my loved ones and they want to help me but don't know what to do for the best. I tell them to do this and then I tell them to undo what they just did. I tell them I need this and then tell them I don't. It's mayhem of the first order when I have a full blown Sickle Cell crisis.

I want to tell them that I will be okay but can't find the words to say so, because of the agonizing pain that is going through my body. And so, I watch them as they panic, are distressed with me, cry with me, pray for me and are just there for me.

Of course I have others who are super cool and will just take it in their stride because they don't want me to see them unable to cope as I am most certainly not coping. I mean it would not be a good thing for all of us to be crying because of one person's pain would it?

I have always described a Sickle Cell crisis as a hurricane, it can start suddenly, bring a lot of devastation to one's body and just leave just as suddenly, just like that when it is ready to depart. And guess what, it leaves my physical body with the devastating after effects.

I sometimes wonder about the damage, those crises had wrecked on my body and it does take time to get back to normal again. One thing I have noticed with Sickle Cell, is one can never get used to the deadly pain. It is impossible to bear the pain because the pain is so unbearable that one wants to die, I have prayed to God to kill me right there and then in the middle of a crisis several times over.

How can one's body go through such mutilation and still function afterwards like nothing happened to it? How can one go through days or weeks of agonizing pain and psychologically remain the same? How? But that is what every warrior who has a crisis does; after the wreckage, we dust ourselves up and we keep it moving.

To all those who have seen me sick over the years, from when I was small to now and helped me one way or another, I would like to say thank you to you all.

Sickle Cell and Hearing the Voice of God

I was under the weather last month and thank goodness I am back on my feet and facing the world squarely. The interesting thing about the situation I found myself in was I did not have a crisis per se as I always have pains in one part of my body or another but just get on with life; I don't like pity parties. However, if I did not have a divine intervention, who knows what would have happened?

Thanks be to God because without me hearing that still small voice telling me to go to the pain clinic, I would not have made my way to the hospital, after all living with pain is common and regular in the life of someone with Sickle cell. On arrival to the pain clinic, after the blood tests, I was told by the doctor that my iron, oxygen and my blood levels were all very low.

When someone has insufficient red blood cells or the ones they have do not work properly, the body is left short of the oxygen it needs to function and this is where the name anemia was coined from. Vitamin-deficiency anemia is when there are low levels of nutrients, such as vitamins B12 or folic acid in one's diet. These anemias change the shape of red blood cells, which makes them less effective.

People with Sickle cell produce less red blood cells and their body destroys red blood cells faster than they can be made. Complications due to low oxygen is when one's oxygen level is lower than normal, one could get hypoxemia or hypoxia, so my doctor tells me.

He continued that without oxygen, my brain, liver, and other organs can be damaged just minutes after symptoms start. Blood carries oxygen to the cells throughout your body and keep them healthy.

Another difficulty that could arise because of low iron could be depression, heart problems (if you do not have enough hemoglobin carrying red blood cells, your heart has to work harder to move oxygen-rich blood through your body. Cells in tissues need a steady supply of oxygen to work well. Typically, hemoglobin in red blood cells takes up oxygen in the lungs and carries it to all the tissues of the body. When one's heart has to work harder, this can lead to several conditions: irregular heartbeats, heart murmur, an enlarged heart or even heart failure).

Other complications could be increased risk of infections (people diagnosed with Sickle cell are prone to a higher level of infection) or even motor or cognitive development delay in children. Treatment of iron-deficiency is dependent on the cause severity of the condition.

Once I got better, I went back to eating and drinking one of my self-made drinks that I currently love making; and here is the recipe: infusing hibiscus leaves, fresh mint leaves, fresh ginger, fresh beetroots, fresh lemons, cloves, star anise, juniper berries in hot water and drink a glass a day. Everything in this super healthy drink will help people with Sickle cell. I'm using what is available where I live but you can also create your own drink; essentials ingredients could be the following, namely: hibiscus tea, moringa, beetroots and water.

Sickle Cell and Poetry

Having SCD is so horrible, especially when one has a crisis. I know that over the years, I have tried to not have anyone around when I am sick because my loved ones can't cope seeing me in so much pain. Pain of any sort cannot be shared and all what the other party can do is say sorry. David O and I have tried to write a poem about pain.

Different sounds that we make, when we are in pain; that pain of vaso-occlusive crisis that occurs in sickle cell warriors. Sometimes, it is the sound of the pain of a pregnant woman in labor; at her term of pregnancy, in her active labor; groaning, crying, screaming in agony; trying to push harder for her baby's delivery; sweating profusely and crying deeply, the sounds of labor pains can also be that of someone having a sickle cell crisis.

Sometimes, it is the sound of gasping for breath; experienced by someone having an asthma attack; as the chest is too stiffened to let out air; and the body is too blue to hold in air; the gasping is a sound of pain, the deep soreness that requires deep labored breathing.

Oh God, take this pain away; it's either the pain goes or you take me; there is no way that I can survive this pain; come 'on Lord, do something quick;' I can feel that I am going to die; I can't hear or sense or feel God. I am disoriented with aches and losing the will to live.

Where is the pain, I hear them ask? My back, chest, legs, shoulders, ribs, arms, knees, joints, thigh, shin, lower back; my whole body is in anguish; how can I endure this ferocious pain, surging through my entire body? How can I? Surely, my body can't cope because this is mind-blowing agony.

I'm being asked, is it acute or chronic? I'm having a crisis and I need to have a dictionary to describe the pain I am going through? Can the questions come later please? I need help right here and right now. No questions, just bombard my body with the injections because I can't handle this level of pain.

Sickle cell pain, give me a break; not you again; I'm off to celebrate at a party in a few hours' time and you rear your ugly head? No way, you will not spoil my joy today, you so won't. I will not allow you to spoil things for me as you always do. You did the same nonsense when I was sitting for my exams some months back, I will not allow you to steal my joy.

My back hurts like no man's business, these tablets are not working. Can I get you to put a box of books on my back? Yes? No? They think I am mad; am I? No, I am not! But I am in pain, in distress and need to deal with this chronic and acute pain, so, where is that heavy suitcase again? Ok, you found it, just put this heavy load on my back. Phew! Slow relief.

Nobody knows the source of my pain and when I choose to tell them I get 'aww'; don't aww me; I am a survivor. A victor and a warrior. Some people didn't make it through their last crisis, I did, painful as it was. I'm alive and will shout from the rooftop that it is well. No, it isn't Tola, don't lie; I am not lying though, right now, minimal sickle cell pain, it is well.

Sickle cell crisis, I describe it as a hurricane that ravages my body and turns it inside out and outside in with no regard for me, the sitting tenant of this body. Do I spend my time hating you or do I embrace you?

I have decided to ignore you and keep living my life the best that I can, knowing that I'll have painful days, good days, bad days, off days and pain free days all depending on the severity of the pain.

How can you describe an existence of pain? People see you and they admire you; they say you are strong; they say you are a warrior; they say you are a survivor. All lovely words but would they think I am strong if they saw me sick, screaming, crying my eyes out, wimping, curling up, twisting or writhing in pain? What would they say? Would they stay or would they leave me?

I am in pain and you don't get me; you think my issues are too much but I'm in pain. The pain is driving me crazy; I can't think straight, I don't know what I want. Yes, I told you to get me some water and now I don't want the water anymore. Don't be irritated, it's just that I can't see an end to this hellhole that I am currently in, pain wise.

My exam is today; I barely slept all night. I have been studying hard for months for today and now this? Who do I call? Who do I tell? Are they going to believe me? After all, my friends and I were studying together till midnight and about 2am this unwanted, unwelcome SC crisis starts, without my say so shows up. I am gutted.

No matter what your pain is like, It is an agonizing pain, it's severe pain, its soft tissue pain, it's acute pain, it's excruciating pain, it's chronic pain, it's ferocious pain; it's bone pain, it's aching pain, it's throbbing pain, its breakthrough pain; it's intense pain, it's referred pain; it's piercing pain, it's unbearable pain, it's hurting pain, it's uncomfortable pain, it's phantom pain or it's total pain. The moans and groans we make, are various sounds uttered from the soul of a survivor, a warrior yearning for freedom, who wants to be free from the pain of sickle cell anemia.

Sickle Cell and the Process of Blood Exchange

A couple of years ago, I had to go for a deep compression surgery on my left shoulder, due to one of the complications of Sickle cell, avascular necrosis (AVN). Owing to sickle cell, no surgery is straight forward and any surgery (big or small), is a big deal in the life of someone with sickle cell because of various complications that could occur during and after surgery. As such, before the main surgery, I had to have a procedure of blood exchange, which itself is a big deal.

A week before the deep compression surgery, I had to go into hospital early for the blood exchange procedure that lasted a few hours. I got there early and they started preparing the machine that was going to do this huge work of removing my blood and inputting 'good' blood in me.

I was eventually told to lay on the bed and the nurse told me they would have to put a tube into my thigh; I said no and told her I wanted them to look for veins in my hands. Fast forward an hour later, they had poked and pricked me all over my arms (the two nurses were very patient) and there was no vein that could withstand the extracting of blood into the machine.

To say that I was bruised, in a state, upset, and annoyed (at my veins), was an understatement. The thing is I totally detest needles and by this time, I had worked myself into an emotional frenzy. In short as a result of all this, we wasted an hour, actually I did. I was not looking forward to having my thigh cut in order for blood to have to go in but this is the blood exchange procedure.

Once we all decided that this exchange had to happen through my thigh, an ultrasound was brought over, in order to make sure that they knew, where to cut, as the veins and arteries are next to each other and similar. The specialist nurse doing the cutting had to make sure she knew where she was cutting into.

A femoral line is a cannula (tube), is inserted into the femoral vein near the groin, this is what is used to give one the donor blood. It is larger than a cannula that is often used for drips. Due to the fact, that a large vein is required for blood exchange, this involved a specially trained nurse to do this procedure. This is called an automated exchange transfusion.

I had to be given two local anesthetic in order for them to numb the area and this helped because of the small cut to my thigh. Finally after small screams and grunts from yours truly, the tube was in. I was worked up by it all and by this time, I could feel myself being sick but I had to reign my emotions in.

The nurses on duty in this unit, where it was all about giving people blood were very kind, patient and professional. The bags (blood) were changed every so often and by the end of it all, I had been given six bags of blood, (about 10 pints), while my blood that was being extracted was in one big bag. As the bags were being changed, the nurses did their usual observations in order to ascertain, that all was well with me.

When the final bag bleeped alerting me/them that it had finished, I had to be given another local anesthetic in order for them to numb the area before they took the tube out; my goodness, what a palaver (all for a good cause of course).

I asked the nurse why I had to endure another needle prick and why could they not give me the injection intravenously. She said if they did not do so, the patient would have a cardiac arrest and so it had to be a under the skin tissue. I was asking questions and learning so much this day. I wanted to make sure that I tell you this story with all the information I received.

The whole process took about two hours. Once the tube was taken out, my hands and thigh were sore and I was quite tired. They then dressed it all up and lectured me on post-care of the wound. The nurses told me to sit for a while. After I was told to walk around in order for them to observe that my walking was okay. After they bid me good bye but not before giving me a card with a number to call, if I started losing blood (in my mind, I was rejecting that). They also made sure that they gave me various plasters to dress the wound.

When I got home, I ate the sandwich, drink, and fruit that I had been given in hospital (truthfully, I was surprised, as I thought, I was not there long enough to be given anything to eat). But apparently, if you are in any day unit, as a patient, you will be given a light lunch. I took some pain killers and went to bed. It was only early afternoon but it had been such a long day for me. The operation was the following week and I'll talk about it next.

People always ask me the difference between a blood transfusion and a blood exchange. I will discuss both at length further on.

Sickle Cell and Avascular Necrosis Operation – Part 1

The non-stop constant pain started in August 2017. I initially took the pain in my stride and kept on living my life. But by the beginning of the year 2018, the pain was unrelenting and affecting my day to day living in so many ways.

Having problems in the bone joints is called osteonecrosis or avascular necrosis and it is a disease caused by the reduced blood flow to bones in the joints; or it is the death of bone tissue due to a lack of blood supply.

By the time I had surgery, my life was not the same because gradually I could not carry anything heavy whatsoever. Going food shopping became a difficult thing for me. Writing also became an ordeal and sleeping at night became an unpleasant and painful situation because once I laid down, the pain was intensified and unbearable, keeping me awake all night. Lifting a filled up kettle was becoming a nightmare.

My handwriting was becoming illegible. I also started having difficulties with opening cans or twisting a bottle cap. Trying to reach out or lift something was also difficult because I could not stretch my arms very far out. And if I drove long distance, I would suffer the consequences at night. Basically, I would feel the consequence of overdoing anything at night. Like I said, this situation was affecting my day to day living hell but I still kept going.

During the course of that year, I wondered how my old age was going to be? If I was going to be an invalid? If I was going to be crippled? I had so many questions and truth be told, I was scared. I just kept on praying to God to have mercy on me.

Now, the type of surgery that I was going to have is not a big deal but due to Sickle cell, it became one. A healthy person without Sickle cell would go in on the day, very early have the operation and come out later that day.

But due to SC, I was told to arrive the day before, in order that I could be monitored and be put on a drip before surgery. On the day I was going into hospital, I had two brothers in Christ, lovely people come with me to hospital and they stayed chatting with me for a while, which took my mind off things, thanks guys.

When we got to the hospital and ward, I was taken into an en-suite room where I would be before surgery. I was so glad not to be in a ward! The junior doctor came over to put a cannula in. He tried as much as he could after pricking and looking for a vein several times before he found a vein and put the cannula in. I was skeptical about what he had done but because I had friends with me, I wanted him to hurry up and go, so I could keep talking and laughing with my friends.

I was comfortable, I had both a personal nurse and health care assistant looking after me, and this meant whenever I needed something, someone would be there. A doctor from the orthopedic team came to see me and explained the procedure I would be having and he also talked about what could go wrong. In my mind, I was rejecting all the negative things he was saying.

When the night staff started their shift, it was now time for the drip to be put in and of course no water flowed into my veins. I knew the cannula that junior doctor had put in would not work. Anyway, that night, the hunt for veins took another turn until a specialist nurse was called. She started by 'playing the piano' on my arm. I thought to myself, this is interesting and so I asked her what she was doing, she replied that she was looking for a vein and that a lot of medical people did not know about the art of looking for a vein. I kept thinking ok let's see what happens next and truly, after playing with my hand for a couple of minutes, she found a vein.

I was told to drink as much as I could from when I was admitted till 2 am and after I needed to be nil mouth. I did as I was told because this surgery had to be successful; the last two years had been agonising for me. Due to the injection and drip drama, I hardly slept that night and slowly, dawn broke and I was still awake.

The same doctor from the orthopedic team came to see me again first thing and he explained the procedure to me one more time. After he left, the anesthetist also came round to explain what they would be doing too. I appreciated being carried along in terms of being told what was going to happen.

When the orthopedic doctor arrived, one of my sister friends also arrived and heard all what he had to say, this was about 7 am. Around 9.35 am, I was wheeled away for surgery. I was taken to a room with two anesthetics doctors attending to me as they explained what they were going to be doing. I was told that they were going to put an injection in my neck, as they needed to numb the whole shoulder area and the other would be somewhere else (sorry can't remember where).

I was busy watching them and the next thing I knew, I asked a nurse when would I be having surgery and she replied it was all done and I was in the recovery room. I was like what, that was fast! I looked at a clock against the wall and it was about 11.30 am. I was back in my room in time for lunch.

Post-surgery, I noticed I could not lift that hand, no sensation at all, it was numb, my goodness, it was heavy and my arm was in a sling and the shoulder was heavily bandaged up. I was numb from my neck and the anesthetics doctors had told me it would take about 18 hours for the effects to wear off and that was what happened. It only started wearing off after 18 hours but it took longer to feel my shoulder.

After surgery and I was back in my room, sometimes in the afternoon, the same orthopedic doctor came round and told me the operation was successful. Amen somebody! Glory to God.

My friends were with me that evening once again. I was given a lot of morphine in order to numb the pain since it was bone surgery. I was encouraged to drink plenty of water, which I did.

Sickle Cell and Avascular Necrosis
Part 2

I wrote about having had arthroscopy of the shoulder, it was an avascular necrosis surgery for short but you know that the component of medical terminology have these terms that make one fearful. In the first part, I wrote about going into hospital, being admitted and having the surgery and the surgery being successful. So let's continue this story.

The next day after surgery, still in hospital, I started feeling better and made it known to the nurse looking after me, that I was well enough and would like to go home because if the surgery was done on a healthy person, they would have gone home the same day.

Another doctor from the orthopedic team, came to do the rounds with other doctors later in the afternoon and told me I will be allowed to leave that day. Hurray!!! Subsequently, someone from the physiotherapy team came round, asked questions, showed me how to remove the sling and put it back on. She equally showed me hand an arm exercises that I needed to do three times a day. She said I would get a letter from the physio team for an appointment with them in some weeks' time.

As, the medical team, were preparing for me to be discharged from hospital, the nurse looking after me came over that afternoon and gave me a letter for my next post-surgery appointment with the orthopedic team and another letter to give to the nurse at my doctor's practice. Home sweet home, I thought, I will be leaving soon. By this time, I was ready to be discharged, as it was about 4.30 pm but it did not happen until about 7 pm that evening. Yes, I am sure you must be wondering why?

My question exactly; well, it was because I had to wait for the pharmacist to dispense the tablets that I was to take home with me.

Due to issues of substance misuse, there is a rigorous check when it comes to dispensing opioid tablets like morphine and codeine in hospitals now. When used incorrectly, opioid medication can be dangerous because a higher dose can slow one's breathing and one's heart rate, which could lead to death.

The surgery I had was one where 3 holes were drilled into my shoulder joints, (front and back) the method used is keyhole surgery. The procedure is afterwards, blood would start to flow through the bones again and have easy flow. This would in turn stop the bones from collapsing and dying but most importantly, I would eventually be able to use the hand without any limitations again. Lord, I am so thankful!

In people with healthy bones, new bone is always replacing old bones. In osteonecrosis, the lack of blood flow causes the bone to break down faster than the body can make enough new bones. One can have osteonecrosis in one or several bone joints. It is most common in the upper leg, upper arm, knees, shoulder and ankles. This can affect men and women of any age, but it usually strikes on one's thirties, forties and fifties.

It is one of the many complications of Sickle Cell Anemia. Prior to surgery, the symptoms were getting worse, I was unable to bend, move or use my arms, hands as I used to. Mostly, my day to day living was dwindling and I was becoming incapacitating. In my case, sleeping became unbearable, as I would toss and turn all night, because the pains were in both shoulders and it affected whatever side I slept on.

Many people have no symptoms in the early stages of avascular necrosis. As the condition worsens, one's affected joint might hurt only when one puts weight on it. Eventually, one might feel the pain all the time, and even when one is lying down. Pain can be mild or severe and usually develops gradually. Pain associated with avascular necrosis of the hip, will centre on the groin, thigh or buttock. Some people develop avascular necrosis on both sides (bilateral) such as both hips, either knees or shoulders.

I took time out after surgery to recover and get all the morphine out of my system and after 3 weeks, I was back on my feet. People asked me after a week, if I feel different with the arm in question and I did not feel any different, as it was too early to notice any difference. I think the reason why I didn't feel any difference at the early stage was because despite my inability to do a lot of what I used to do in the past, I still pushed myself and used my arms.

My body is used to being hit by a tornado, once in a while, (I mean having a sickle cell crisis) and it is used to getting up after the hurricane and keeping things moving. I am used to doing more with less, health wise all throughout my life.

Post-surgery, I did not carry any heavy stuff, I tried to not use that arm, as I am still giving it time to heal; I went to the nurse to remove the stitches after 10 days and the wounds had both healed nicely. I also had an appointment with the physio team and I was made to do some exercises there and told to continue them at home. They want me to continue to see them because they want to help me build strength back into my arms.

I am thankful to God for His goodness over me. There is no such thing as an inconsequential surgery because something could go wrong at any point in time, from the moment one is given the anesthetic drug that is injected into one's body, in order to numb a large area of the body, to the surgery itself.

So if you had successful surgeries over the years, and it was successful, be thankful. Let's not take it for granted because some people had the same operation you and I had and did not make it through.

I would like to thank everyone who was with me, physically, spiritually and emotionally through this journey of mine, much love.

Sickle Cell and Years 2010-2019

I thought I would reflect on this disease called Sickle Cell anemia and how it has affected me in the last decade. To be frank with you, Sickle cell affected me more this decade than all other decades. I look back and remember how at a time I had three jobs going (I was working at the BBC, I was sitting as a magistrate and I was working as a counsellor) and Sickle Cell was not a factor that I considered in anything that I did, simply because it was kept in the background. Don't get me wrong, of course I fell ill, got up and kept on working.

As this decade started, I decided to relocate back home to Lagos, in Nigeria and be with my elderly mother. To be honest, I had no consideration for Sickle Cell, when making plans to move back home. I mean, I had been living and working abroad for such a long time and had been able to hold down three jobs at a go, so what is Sickle cell? I therefore did not give it any attention when I made plans to relocate. I was trying to adjust to living in Lagos and getting things in place, I am talking about my comforts, anything to help me not to fall ill.

At the best of times, Lagos or Nigeria as a whole is stressful and I so wasn't used to the stresses I encountered; it was on another level. Long story short, I invariably fell ill, had a crisis and we thought it was going to be a small thing but days went by and I was getting worse. In the end, I had no choice but to be taken to a private hospital.

I was on admission for a week and I would just like to pause my story and thank my lovely big cousins SS, my cousin Lawunmi and my mother who were with me day and night. I also want to thank my other cousins and uncles as well; you are all the best.

After a week, I was discharged and it was only then that I realised that I had gone blind in my left eye! I was totally chagrined, terrified and pissed off; what is this, I asked myself? It was not a pleasant experience and so I researched about it and found out, this can be a Sickle cell complication, called 'Sickle cell retinopathy or retinal hemorrhage'. Here I was, once again, learning something new about this disease that I was diagnosed it.

In my human mind, I thought it must have been brought on by the stress of being sick and relocation; hoping, praying that my vision would go back to normal soon however a few weeks by and I still could not see with my left eye.

It became a situation whereby I was advised I needed to go and see an ophthalmologist in Lagos. I was like, what! I just could not comprehend what was going on. Finally, I decided, I needed to come back to my base London and see doctors who know me, know about Sickle cell and doctors I trusted.

I then came back and it was then I truly understood the expression 'home is where the heart is'. At this junction, I would like to thank 'my mum' in London, who took me in and blessed me by looking after me and praying over me. I started going to my hematology clinic, was referred to one of the main eye hospitals in London.

In due course, the blood vessels started to clear; it was like peeling an onion in order to get to its core, and after about eight months of petrifying moments, wondering if I would ever see again from my left eye, the whole thing cleared and my vision was restored and now my eyesight is back to normal.

I had so many other incidents of Sickle cell complications and the most recent one was AVN (Avascular necrosis: death of the bone), that started about two years ago and was affecting my shoulders and knees. Again, I had to be strong for me until I had the operation and now the pains have subsided and it feels good to be able to do the day to day things I was unable to do as the situation got worse.

In this last decade, I have also met some Sickle cell warriors and some of you have been brave enough to share their story through my weekly column in Punch newspaper. As I have read some personal stories, I thought to myself that here I was bemoaning my lot, thinking I had it tough but some people have it tougher and for that I would like to salute all the Sickle cell warriors who read this column and also friends of warriors who get in touch or pass the column on.

Can I just encourage all Sickle cell warriors to not give up and to keep fighting this personal battle of yours? I believe in Kingdom connections and so my hope for you, in the next decade is that you will be sent people or that special person who would love you for you and you would not have to lie about who you are.

You are special, Sickle cell or not; Sickle cell sets you apart, that is for sure but it is for a better outcome because people can see you or read about you and point at you saying, that you are an inspiration to others who have nothing wrong with them.

PART 2: VITAMINS, MINERALS and MACRONUTRIENTS

All vitamins are identified as key nutrients: the body cannot produce them and so they must be obtained through diet; minerals are similarly identified as key nutrients. Vitamins and minerals are equally essential for the healthy functioning of the body.

Although they are all considered micronutrients, vitamins and minerals differ in basic ways. Vitamins are organic and can be broken down by heat, air, or acid. Minerals are inorganic and hold on to their chemical structure.

So the difference between vitamins and minerals are that minerals are inorganic. Calcium, potassium, zinc, selenium, those are minerals. Vitamins are organic materials, so either plants or animals make vitamins. For instance, vitamin D or vitamin E or vitamin C, you've heard of vitamin C coming from oranges, well oranges make vitamin C out of chemicals they get out of the soil.

Humans produce vitamin D from sunlight shining on your skin, and there's a chemical reaction that allows you to produce vitamin D. Or you can get vitamin D through supplementation.

Sickle Cell and Vitamins

Vitamins help to regulate chemical reactions in the body. There are 13 vitamins, including vitamins A, B complex, C, D, E, and K. Because most vitamins cannot be made in the body, we must obtain them through consumption. Many people say that they feel more energetic after consuming vitamins, but vitamins are not a source of energy (calories). Vitamins are best consumed through a varied diet and taking supplements if necessary.

Nowadays, we are told to eat plant foods and these are: beans, peas, lentils, fruit, vegetable, whole grains, nuts and seeds; these are plant proteins. We are also encouraged to increase the diversity of what we eat and to not eat the same kind of food every day.

Eating colourful vegetables and fruits every day can have a great effect on cutting down on the risk of illness. Each coloured fruit or vegetable has a unique set of disease fighting chemicals and the best way to benefit from them is to eat a rainbow coloured diet and eat vegetables in season.

Try to minimize your consumption of processed foods, refined foods and fast food. Include the likes of sweet potatoes and Omega-3 fish into your diet; cook with olive oil, sunflower oil, ground nut oil or coconut oil if you are able to do so.

Drink herbal teas, or white, green teas instead of coffee; drink more water; fresh fruit juices; water with lemon; mint or cucumber; ginger with water; ginger and lemon with water etc throughout the day.

There is a theory out there about fixing one's eating habit. Most of us eat from daybreak till sundown; meaning one is eating for a period of over sixteen hours.

Apparently, eating in such a manner does not allow one's body to align itself to the food being eaten. It is said that if one shortens the window of time that one eats, then this could boost one's overall health and people have reported improved energy, better sleep and weight loss.

The study is that our bodies are designed to digest and absorb food more efficiently during a relatively short period of time each day. The body then repairs itself and burns stored fat when we fast. It's about thinking about eating over a period of twelve hours, ten or nine hours a day. Say you start eating from 8am till 8pm, you could reduce it from 9am to 8pm or 9am to 7pm. If at night you are hungry after 8 or 9pm, then just drink water or any of what I have mentioned above and snack on nuts for example.

Patients with SC anemia have greater than average requirements for both calories and micro-nutrients. A diet emphasising fruits, vegetables, whole grains and legumes will provide a greater proportion of essential nutrients than a typical Western diet. And suitable supplementation (1-3 times of the recommended intakes for most essential nutrients) can prevent deficient and may decrease the likelihood of disease exacerbation.

Anyone who suffers from Sickle Cell Anemia, will need to make a conscious effort to eat well and take some supplements. On a personal note, I prefer to eat food that contain the vitamins that my body needs. You will need a high calorie, nutrient dense diet and adequate fluid consumption to maintain hydration.

The most essential vitamins to take, food wise are:

Vitamin A and carotenoids

Vitamin A is a fat-soluble vitamin that is necessary for the proper function of the immune system, vision, and cell growth. It acts as an antioxidant in cells and helps repair damage.

We need vitamin A for healthy skin and mucus membranes, our immune system, good eye health and vision. Vitamin A can be sourced from the food we eat, through beta carotene, for example, or in supplement form.

Carotenoids are plant pigments responsible for bright red, yellow and orange hues in many fruits and vegetables. They also have an important anti-oxidant function of deactivating free radicals - single oxygen atoms that can damage cells by reacting with other molecules.

Some carotenoids are converted by the body to vitamin A, which is essential to vision, and normal growth and development. Carotenoids also have anti-inflammatory and immune system benefits. It also helps ward off age-related macular degeneration (AMD), a leading cause of vision loss.

Vitamin A is found in foods like Apricots, asparagus, beef liver, meat, fish, dairy products, beetroots, broccoli, carrots, corn, guava, kale, mangoes, carrots, apricots spinach, all greens, nectarines, peaches, pink grapefruit, pumpkin, sweet potatoes, red peppers, broccoli, tangerines, tomatoes and watermelon.

Vitamin B1 (Thiamine or Thiamin)

Vitamin B1, or thiamine, is a vitamin that the body requires for energy metabolism and for cell growth, function, and development.

Thiamine is also necessary for the proper function of the brain. It is found in meat, fish, and whole grains. Breakfast cereals are often fortified with vitamin B1.

Vitamin B2 (Riboflavin)

Vitamin B2, or riboflavin, is a vitamin that the body needs to produce energy and facilitate cell growth, function, and development. It is also used to metabolize drugs and fats. The vitamin is bright yellow. It is found in organ meats, (there are many different types of organ meat, including liver, tongue, heart and kidneys), eggs, milk, lean meats, and vegetables. Cereals and some grains are fortified with riboflavin.

Vitamin B3 (Niacin)

Vitamin B3, or niacin, is a B vitamin that the body uses to convert food into energy and store it. It also aids the function of nerves and promotes the health of the skin, tissues, and digestive system. Niacin is found in milk, eggs, canned tuna, lean meats, fish, peanuts, legumes, and poultry and enriched cereals and breads.

Vitamin B 6

Vitamin B6, also known as pyridoxine, helps the body to use and store energy from protein and carbohydrates in food form hemoglobin, the substance in red blood cells that carries oxygen around the body. Vitamin B6 is a B vitamin that is needed for more than 100 different reactions in the body.

It is critical for proper brain function, to manufacture neurotransmitters, and it helps regulate mood. Good sources of this vitamin include beef liver, lean meat, legumes, fish, leafy greens, starchy vegetables like potatoes, and fruits (excluding citrus fruit). Fortified cereals have the vitamin, too.

Vitamin B6 is found in a wide variety of foods, including: pork, poultry, such as chicken or turkey, fish, bread (sour bread or fortified - which are better for your stomach), wholegrain cereals, such as oatmeal, wheat germ and brown rice, eggs, vegetables, soya beans, peanuts, milk, potatoes and some fortified breakfast cereals.

Vitamin B12

Vitamin B12, or cobalamin, is a vitamin that helps you break down food for energy. Your body uses it to form red blood cells and DNA. You also need it for proper neurological function and to make SAMe, a compound your body needs to make genetic material, proteins, hormones, and fats. Vitamin B12 is found in clams, liver, fortified cereal, fish, meat, dairy products, and eggs.

Vitamin C

Vitamin C (also termed ascorbic acid) is an antioxidant vitamin that your body needs to maintain healthy bones, skin and muscles. It's well known for being a potent antioxidant, as well as having positive effects on skin health and immune function. It is a water-soluble vitamin that's found in many foods, particularly fruits and vegetables. It's also vital for collagen synthesis, which supports skin integrity as one ages, connective tissue, bones, teeth and your small blood vessels.

The human body cannot produce or store vitamin C. Therefore, it's essential to consume it regularly in sufficient amounts. Foods rich in vitamin C include broccoli, rose hip is a small, sweet, tangy fruit from the rose plant. It's loaded with vitamin C. Approximately six rose hips provide 119 mg of vitamin C, chilli peppers, guava, blackcurrants, kiwi, thyme, parsley, kale (spinach, greens), brussel sprouts, cauliflower, kale, spinach, orange juice (fresh), lemon, sweet potato, lychees, red or yellow peppers, papaya, strawberries, oranges, broccoli, and other types of fruits and veggies.

Most people easily get enough vitamin C in their daily diets. Vitamin C is a water-soluble vitamin so you need to eat vitamin C rich foods regularly or take a supplement to make sure you always maintain adequate levels.

Vitamin D

Vitamin D is a fat-soluble vitamin that the body needs to regulate cell growth, combat inflammation, and enhance immune function. Vitamin D works with calcium to maintain strong, healthy bones and help prevent osteoporosis.

Good sources of vitamin D include fatty fish like salmon, mackerel, and tuna. Smaller amounts are found in egg yolks. Fortified milk and orange juice may contain vitamin D as well. The best way to get vitamin D is to spend approximately 10-15 minutes outside in the sun on a clear day without sunscreen. Your skin manufactures vitamin D when you get sun exposure.

Vitamin E

Vitamin E is an antioxidant vitamin that protects cells against free radicals. Free radicals may be produced by things that can harm cells and tissues including pollution, cigarette smoke, sunlight, and more. Vitamin E is a group of powerful antioxidants that protect your cells from oxidative stress. Adequate vitamin E levels are essential for the body to function normally. If you don't get enough, you may become more prone to infections, experience impaired eyesight or suffer from muscle weakness. Fortunately, vitamin E is widespread in foods.

As a result, you are unlikely to become deficient unless your nutrient absorption is impaired. Nevertheless, everyone should try to eat plenty of whole foods rich in vitamin E. Good sources of vitamin E include wheat germ oil, sunflower seeds, almonds, hazelnuts, and peanuts. Nut butters are good sources of vitamin E. Some people are allergic to nuts, cashew nuts, pecan nuts.

Smaller amounts of vitamin E are found in safflower oil, sunflower oil, broccoli, leafy vegetables, and spinach. Salmons, goose meat, avocado, red raw pepper, mangoes, snails, crayfish, cod, trout, pistachio, pumpkin seeds.

Vitamin K

Vitamin K is a nutrient that is necessary to maintain healthy bones. It serves as a co-enzyme, or a necessary helper, for the production of proteins that aid in both blood clotting and bone metabolism. Vitamin K is found in abundance in leafy vegetables like collards, turnip greens, spinach, and kale. It is also found in broccoli.

Smaller amounts are found in soy, carrot juice, canned pumpkin, pomegranate juice, and okra. The best natural source of vitamin K that has the greatest amount of this vitamin is a fermented soybean dish, otherwise known as natto.

Folic Acid

Folic acid is the man-made version of the vitamin folate (also known as vitamin B9). Folate helps the body make healthy red blood cells and is found in certain foods.

Some cereals and other foods are fortified with a form of the vitamin called folic acid. Folate is a B vitamin. Natural sources are found in green leafy vegetables, nuts, meat, poultry, beans, fruit, seafood, eggs, grains, liver, spinach, asparagus and brussels sprouts.

Sickle Cell and Minerals

Minerals are components of foods that are involved in many body functions. For example, calcium and magnesium are important for bone structure, and iron is needed for our red blood cells to transport oxygen. Like vitamins, minerals are not a source of energy and are best obtained through a varied diet and supplements if necessary.

Calcium

Calcium is a critical mineral that helps make up your teeth and bones. It is also necessary for muscle contractions, including the proper functioning of the heart. Daily calcium requirements differ due to your age and gender. Some groups of people are at risk for having inadequate calcium levels.

Good food sources of calcium include milk, yogurt, and cheese. Broccoli and green leafy vegetables like kale also have calcium. Sardines and salmon with bones supply calcium. So do calcium-fortified orange juice and cereal. Ask your doctor if you should take a calcium supplement. If you take any medications, ask your doctor or pharmacist whether or not calcium supplements interact with anything you are taking.

Iron

Iron is a mineral that is critical in the body because it is a constituent of hemoglobin, the protein that carries oxygen from the lungs and delivers it to tissues. You need enough iron to make healthy red blood cells.

A lack of iron causes a condition called iron deficiency anemia. This condition makes you tired because tissues do not receive enough oxygen. Women who are pregnant and those who have heavy menstrual cycles have greater requirements for iron.

The best sources of iron include fortified breakfast cereal, oysters, white beans, dark chocolate, and beef liver. Smaller amounts are found in spinach, lentils, kidney beans, sardines, and chickpeas. If you take an iron supplement, take it with a little vitamin C or vitamin C-rich food because this nutrient boosts the absorption of the mineral.

Magnesium

Mineral that our bodies rely on to feel fit, healthy and full of vitality. Magnesium is also required for the formation of bones, muscles, contractions and blood pressure regulation. Magnesium helps promote energy, sleep, blood sugar and hormone balance.

Magnesium is found in a variety of food, but the best sources tend to be green leafy vegetables (spinach, kale, etc); raw cacao; nuts and seeds; fruits (figs, avocado, bananas, raspberries); legumes (black beans, chickpeas, kidney beans); seafood (salmon, mackerel, tuna); whole grains (brown rice, oats); raw avocado, dark chocolate, tofu, baked beans, chollera powder.

Omega-3 fatty acids

Promotes brain health, your heart, fights inflammation; can improve bone and joints. Omega-3 fatty acid supplements. These long-chain omega-3 fatty acids increase the fluidity of red blood cell membranes, which may prevent sickle cell crisis. It is good for your skin.

Food rich in Omega-3 are: Oily fish (mackerel, salmon, seabass, sardines, herring, shrimps, trout); Seaweed, nori, spirulina, and chlorella powder, walnuts; kidney beans.

Individuals with SCD are often low in these vitamins and nutrients. These deficiencies cause a significant depreciation in blood-antioxidant status in these patients, and the resulting oxidative stress may precipitate vaso-occlusion crisis or related acute chest syndrome.

Potassium

Potassium is a mineral that serves as an electrolyte in the body. It also regulates blood pressure and kidney function. You need potassium for your heart, brain, and nervous system to work properly. The balance of sodium to potassium in the body is critical for several processes. Potatoes, prunes, sweet potatoes, carrots, bananas, green leafy vegetables, cantaloupe, and tomatoes are good sources of potassium.

Selenium

Selenium is a trace mineral your body needs for proper functioning of the thyroid gland and immune system. It is an antioxidant that protects cells and tissues against free radical damage.

Selenium deficiency is rare. It may occur in regions where selenium content in the soil is low, especially in those who are vegetarian or vegan.

Selenium levels may also be low in those who suffer from HIV and in those who undergo long-term kidney dialysis. Dialysis removes some selenium from the blood. The best food sources of selenium are nuts, seafood, organ meats, meat, and eggs. Whole grains like brown rice and cereals also contain the mineral.

Zinc

Zinc is a mineral that's essential for good health. Zinc is a mineral that is necessary to maintain your senses of taste and smell. It is vital to the immune system and your body needs it for wound healing. Zinc is one of the minerals that helps protect your eyes and keeps vision sharp as you age. Zinc helps blood clots.

It's required for the functions of over 300 enzymes and involved in many important processes in your body. It metabolizes nutrients, maintains your immune system and grows and repairs body tissues. Your body doesn't store zinc, so you need to eat enough every day to ensure you're meeting your daily requirements.

Food rich in Zinc are: meat is an excellent source of zinc. Red meat is a particularly great source, but ample amounts can be found in all different kinds of meat, including beef, lamb and pork. Shellfish (crabs); legumes like chickpeas, lentils and beans all contain substantial amounts of zinc. Seeds; nuts (Eating nuts such as pine nuts, peanuts, cashews and almonds can boost your intake of zinc.).

Dairy foods like cheese and milk provide a host of nutrients, including zinc. Eggs; whole grains like wheat, quinoa, rice and oats contain some zinc. Potatoes and dark chocolate.

Studies indicate supplementation of zinc, magnesium, vitamins A, C, and E or treatment with a combination of high-dose antioxidants can reduce the percentage of irreversibly sickled cells.

If you have SCD, you will need a high calorie, nutrient dense diet and adequate fluid consumption to maintain hydration. The most essential vitamins and nutrients to take are: Vitamins A, B6, C, E, Magnesium, Zinc and Omega-3.

As a matter of fact, when fruits and vegetables are consumed continuously, they help reduce the risk of many health conditions. That is why medical practitioners have been advising that we add fruits and vegetables to our diet because of their health benefits.

The body needs many minerals to function and having too much of one major mineral can result in a deficiency of another. A balanced diet should be able to provide you all the minerals that your body needs.

Sickle and Macronutrients

Patients with SC anemia have greater than average requirements for both calories and micro-nutrients. A diet emphasising fruits, vegetables, whole grains and legumes will provide a greater proportion of essential nutrients than a typical Western diet and appropriate supplementation (1-3 times the recommended intakes for most essential nutrients) can prevent deficiency and may decrease the likelihood of disease exacerbation.

Anti-oxidants

Antioxidant plant phenols, such as flavonoids, may also reduce the oxidative stress in SCD. These long-chain omega-3 fatty acids increase the fluidity of red blood cell membranes, which may prevent sickle cell crisis and have significant therapeutic benefits including reduction of severe anemia.

Antioxidants are compounds produced in your body and found in foods. They help defend your cells from damage caused by potentially harmful molecules known as free radicals. Foods rich in anti-oxidant include, dark chocolate, pecan nuts, strawberry, agabalumo, kale, Ugu, red cabbage, beans, beetroots, spinach (efo), okra, plantain.

Carbohydrates

Carbohydrates can be grouped into two categories: simple and complex. Simple carbohydrates are sugars whereas complex carbohydrates consist of starch and dietary fibre. Carbohydrate is the energy that is used first to fuel muscles and the brain.

Soluble fibre (fruits, legumes, nuts, seeds, brown rice, and oat, barley and rice brans) lowers blood cholesterol and helps to control blood sugar levels. Insoluble fibre are (wheat and corn bran, whole-grain breads and cereals, vegetables, fruit skins, nuts) doesn't provide any calories.

It helps to alleviate digestive disorders like constipation. Sources of carbohydrates include grain products such as breads, cereals, pasta, and rice as well as fruits and vegetables.

Fat

The fat in food includes a mixture of saturated and unsaturated fat. Animal-based foods such as meats and milk products are higher in saturated fat whereas most vegetable oils are higher in unsaturated fat. Compared to carbohydrate and protein, each gram of fat provides more than twice the amount of calories (9 kcal per gram). Nevertheless, dietary fat does play an important role in a healthy diet. Fat maintains skin and hair, cushions vital organs, provides insulation, and is necessary for the production and absorption of certain vitamins and hormones.

Flavonoids

Flavonoids are various compounds found naturally in many fruits and vegetables. They're also in plant products like wine, tea, and chocolate.

There are six different types of flavonoids found in food, and each kind is broken down by your body in a different way. Flavonoids are rich in antioxidant activity and can help your body ward off every day toxins.

Including more flavonoids in your diet is a great way to help your body stay healthy and potentially decrease your risk of some chronic health conditions. Foods: onions, kale, grapes and red wine, tea, peaches, berries, tomatoes, lettuce, broccoli, white tea, green tea, oolong tea, black tea, apples, purple and red grapes, blueberries, strawberries, cocoa and chocolate products, parsley, red peppers, celery, chamomile, peppermint, lemons, limes, oranges, grapefruit, efirin (scent leaves).

Plant phenols

Polyphenols are micronutrients that we get through certain plant-based foods. They're packed with antioxidants and potential health benefits. It's thought that polyphenols can improve or help treat digestion issues. Foods: cloves, cocoa powder, all berries, blackcurrants, cherries (agabalumo), apples, plums, beans, nuts, vegetables, corn, red onions, spinach, black or green tea, red wine, efirin (scent leaves).

Protein

Protein from food is broken down into amino acids by the digestive system. These amino acids are then used for building and repairing muscles, red blood cells, hair and other tissues, and for making hormones.

Adequate protein intake is also important for a healthy immune system. Protein is a source of calories (4 kcal per gram).

Main sources of protein are animal products like meat, fish, poultry, milk, cheese and eggs and vegetable sources like legumes (beans, lentils, dried peas, nuts) and seeds.

Water

Water is a vital nutrient for good health. Most of our body weight (60-70%) is made up of water. Water helps to control our body temperature, carries nutrients and waste products from our cells, and is needed for our cells to function.

It is recommended that adults drink 8 glasses of fluid daily (or more in hot weather or during physical activity). This fluid does not have to be water alone. It can also be obtained from juice, milk, soup, and foods high in water such as fruits and vegetables.

Caffeine-containing beverages (coffee, tea, cola) don't count because caffeine is a diuretic, making us lose water. A great plus for water in comparison to the other fluids is that it hydrates our body without extra calories.

PART 3: FOOD NUTRITIONAL GUIDE

One thing you can do to help yourself if you suffer from Sickle Cell is to eat well and let food be your medicine. By that I mean, eating food that have a lot of nutrients and will help boost your immunity. Food does the following:

1. Decreases Inflammation – Most diseases today are due to inflammation. By reducing inflammation your body is better able to heal from any disease.

2. Alkalizes body – Your body should have an average pH of 7.36. Green vegetable juices like wheat grass and spinach help restore the body's proper pH. By alkalizing your body your cells can heal and regenerate at the highest level.

3. Eliminates Toxins – Toxicity has become epidemic in or society today and is a major cause of our increase in hormonal imbalance and autoimmune diseases.

4. Optimum Nutrients – Many of today's illnesses are due to nutritional deficiencies. Most of the foods we eat today are processed and stripped of all vitamins, minerals, anti-oxidants and enzymes. This diet slows the aging process, improves mental capacity, and increases energy levels.

Sickle Cell and Food to Boost your Immune System

When I was doing my research about what topic to write, I stumbled across this article and thought to share it with you. While proper hygiene i.e. washing your hands often and keeping them away from your nose, mouth, and eyes (which serve as pathways for germs to enter the body) is the best defense against catching a contagious bug, here's what science has to say about supporting a healthy immune system with food.

1. Beans and other foods with prebiotic fibre

Fibre, or carbohydrates that pass through the digestive tract to promote healthy digestion and elimination, is an essential part of a nutritious diet.

Eating prebiotic fibre, a type that helps to feed the healthy bacteria found in your gut, may play a role in supporting immune system functioning. Foods containing prebiotic fibre include beans, onions, leeks, garlic, whole grains (including oats), cashews, soy and fruits such as bananas.

2. Citrus fruits

Oranges, grapefruits, lemons and limes are a great source of vitamin C, a potent antioxidant that plays a role in immune cell functioning (i.e. helps keep your immune system in good shape). That said, peeling a single orange won't do much to prevent you from getting sick or shorten the length of a cold.

Developing a habit of eating a range of foods that contain vitamin C as well as a variety of antioxidants can support overall health, according to a 2017 study review published in the journal *Nutrients*. Researchers also found that vitamin C deficiency is associated with impaired immunity and higher susceptibility to infections.

Another caveat: eating an orange beats drinking a glass of orange juice, since fruit is higher than juice in fibre, antioxidants, phytonutrients and prebiotics, all of which support health.

3. Shellfish and other foods high in zinc

A nutrient that is essential for proper immune system functioning, zinc is found in a whole bunch of tasty foods including oysters (the best source of zinc per serving), mussels and other shellfish, yogurt, milk, poultry, red meat, beans, nuts, ginger, turmeric and wholegrains.

While most people get enough zinc through diet, when you're trying to outrun a virus, supplementing with zinc (at least 75 mg per day) from the onset of a cold until it's gone could help you feel better faster.

The bottom line is if you really want to help the body maintain a healthy immune system, have a diet rich in wholegrains, fresh fruits and vegetables, lean meats, fish, eggs and dairy all year round (particularly during cold and flu season) is vital.

4. Yogurt and other probiotics

The gastrointestinal tract and the trillions of bacteria that live there account for up to 60 percent of the entire immune system, says board-certified gastroenterologist Brittany Seminara, MD, who practices at Atrium Health in Charlotte, North Carolina.

Generally, the guts naturally-occurring bacteria aid in digestion and keep the lining of your gut healthy. However, medications, infections, illness, and other environmental factors (like what you eat) can disturb the balance of gut bacteria: one reason why it may be smart to consume beneficial bacteria known as probiotics, which are available as supplements or in foods like yogurt and fermented foods.

It's also worth repeating: make sure to wash your hands properly (i.e. with soap for at least 20 seconds) and keep them away from your face. Avoid others who are sick, and disinfect places or objects touched by many people (like door handles, phones and keyboards) before using them. Paired with a balanced diet rich in essential nutrients, these habits can help you stay well.

Sickle Cell and Healing Food

If there is a question that I get asked a lot, it is on, what people with Sickle Cell should eat, in order to stay strong and healthy and most especially out of hospital. With Sickle Cell, it is important to eat a well-balanced diet, meaning, your vegetables and fruits.

All the various things and food I recommend, I also do and eat, as staying healthy is very important to me. Even though I look after myself, as much as I can, I still find myself down with a Sickle Cell crisis or something else that would then trigger a Sickle Cell crisis.

During such situations, I wonder if there is more that I should be doing that I did not do. One thing that I have tried to do is – to buy natural food as much as possible. The fresher the food, the better for us. All these genetically modified foods are not good for the human body anyway.

Some countries insist on the labelling of GMO foods but not all countries and such, it is better to buy food labelled 'fresh'. This is about preserving life, living well and the only way that can happen is if you to watch what you are putting inside of you by being more conscious of what you eat as the ultimate goal is not to be admitted into hospital at all or not often.

Medicines are also genetically modified and so, it can sometimes be a losing battle for the human body. And that is the reason why, when I am taking tablets, 8 times out of 10, I will eat some solid food especially if I am indoors. I will not just take tablets on an empty stomach ever.

Sometimes, I might be outside and I feel some pain. This might mean taking my tablets with biscuits or eating crisps. I always have tablets in my bag, for a just in case moment. When I buy crisps, I buy multi-grains crisps and I also tend to eat pop corns more than crisps, as the calories are less and they are more nutritious and now you can buy wholegrain pop corns.

A lot of shops now sell, dried fruits in small pouches; these are worth buying and keeping in your bag. I usually have various nuts, as they are easy to carry in my bag. Please don't misunderstand me, I am not advocating not taking tablets. But I believe in taking tablets with good food, with healthy snacks, like nuts or roasted plantain etc...and not on an empty stomach, especially if you are out an about.

I have compiled a list below, if you don't already eat most of this, then do try to include them in your regular diet.

Healing Foods: all nuts (cashews, almonds, walnuts etc...), all beans, fruits in general, goat milk, butter, coconut oil, olive oil, sesame oil, grapeseed oil, fish oil, all vegetables, eggs, fish, chicken, turkey, lamb, beef, venison, wild game, brown rice, millet, oats, sweet potato, yam, sea salt, apple cider vinegar, balsamic vinegar, herbs and spices, soy sauce (wheat free), honey, maple syrup, purified water, alkanised water, fresh fruit juice, raw lemonade, all manner of spinach, kale, greens, okra, tuna, quinoa, geisha, wheat, brown bread. Red lean meat, liver, seeds (sunflower, sesame), vitamin C, red peppers, broccoli, berries, sardines in a can, boiled eggs, dried figs, beef, kidney beans, dried apricots, corn beef, dates, shrimps, black eyed beans, almonds, raisins, turkey, pork, lamb, cabbage, steak, potatoes (with or without skin), pasta, tomato.

CEREAL: raisin bran, whole wheat, brown bread, gammon, watercress, veal, hot dogs, bagel bread, cereal.

DRINKS: orange, carrot, apple, cherry, grape, cherry, tomato, strawberry juices, red wine, Guinness, V8 drink, pomegranate drink, herbal teas and fermented drinks.

The Healing Foods to consist of eating equal amounts (33% each) of clean protein sources, healthy fats, and low glycemic carbohydrates in the forms of fruits and vegetables.

Of course, with all of this, one can still fall ill and so just take it in your stride. The way I look at it, is at least, I have done all that I can do to look after myself and be healthy and stay out of hospital as much as I can.

Sickle Cell and Alkaline Food

An alkaline diet emphasizes alkaline foods such as whole fruits and vegetables and certain whole grains, which are low in caloric density. Healthy Alkaline Diet Foods involve the ideal balance between acidifying and alkalizing foods.

The body includes a number of organ systems that are adept at neutralizing and eliminating excess acid, but there is a limit to how much acid even a healthy body can cope with effectively. The body is capable of maintaining an acid-alkaline balance provided that the organs are functioning properly, that a well-balanced alkaline diet is being consumed, and that other acid-producing factors, such as tobacco use, are avoided.

A 2012 review published in the *Journal of Environmental Health* found that balancing your body's pH through an alkaline diet can be helpful in reducing morbidity and mortality from numerous chronic diseases and ailments — such as hypertension, diabetes, arthritis, vitamin D deficiency, and low bone density, just to name a few.

How do alkaline diets work? Research shows that diets consisting of highly alkaline foods — fresh vegetables, fruits and unprocessed plant-based sources of protein, for example (peas, beans, kale, grains, nuts, seeds, lentils, spirulina, oats, wild rice, vegetables — result in a more alkaline urine pH level, which helps protect healthy cells and balance essential mineral levels. Alkaline diets (also known as the alkaline ash diets) have been shown to help prevent plaque formation in blood vessels, stop calcium from accumulating in urine, prevent kidney stones, build stronger bones, and more. It is also linked to a longer life expectancy and a quality of life that includes a healthier body and mind.

What Is an Alkaline Diet?

An alkaline diet is one that helps balance the pH level of the fluids in your body, including your blood and urine. Your pH is partially determined by the mineral density of the foods you eat. All living organisms and life forms on earth depend on maintaining appropriate pH levels, and it's often said that disease and disorder cannot take root in a body that has a balanced pH.

Although some experts might not totally agree with this statement, nearly all agree that human life requires a very tightly controlled pH level of the blood of about 7.365–7.4. As *Forbe's Magazine* puts it, "Our bodies go to extraordinary lengths to maintain safe pH levels." Your pH can range between 7.35 to 7.45 depending on the time of day, your diet, what you last ate and when you last went to the bathroom. If you develop electrolyte imbalances and frequently consume too many acidic foods, your body's changing pH level can result in increased "acidosis."

Wondering what exactly "pH level" even means?

What we call pH is short for the potential of hydrogen. It's a measure of the acidity or alkalinity of our body's fluids and tissues. It's measured on a scale from 0 to 14. The more acidic a solution is, the lower its pH. The more alkaline, the higher the number is. A pH of around 7 is considered neutral, but since the optimal human body tends to be around 7.4, we consider the healthiest pH to be one that's slightly alkaline, and pH levels vary throughout the body, with the stomach being the most acidic region.

Even very tiny alterations in the pH level of various organisms can cause major problems. For example, due to environmental concerns, such as increasing CO2 deposition, the pH of the ocean has dropped from 8.2 to 8.1 and various life forms living in the ocean have greatly suffered. The pH level is also crucial for growing plants, and therefore it greatly affects the mineral content of the foods we eat. Minerals in the ocean, soil and human body are used as buffers to maintain optimal pH levels, so when acidity rises, minerals fall.

Examples of Alkaline Vegetables: Beets, Broccoli, Cauliflower, Celery, Cucumber, Kale, Lettuce, Onions, Peas, Peppers, Avocado, Spinach, Tomato.

Examples of Alkaline Fruits: Apple, Banana, Berries, Cantaloupe, Grapes, Melon, Lemon, Orange, Peach, Pear, Watermelon.

Alkaline Protein: Almonds, Chestnuts, Tofu.

Alkaline Spices: Cinnamon, Curry, Ginger, Mustard, Sea Salt, Garlic, Himalayan Salt, real salt.

Alkaline food: pH 9.5 Water, Green drinks, Broccoli, Cabbage, Parsley, Sprouts (alfalfa, bean, pea, soy, etc.), Soy Nuts, (soaked soybeans, then air-dried), Soy lecithin.

Alkaline Diet Benefits

Lowers chronic pain and inflammation: studies have found a connection between an alkaline diet and reduced levels of chronic pain. Chronic acidosis has been found to contribute to chronic back pain, headaches, muscle spasms, menstrual symptoms, inflammation and joint pain.

One study conducted by the society for minerals and trace elements in Germany found that when patients with chronic back pain were given an alkaline supplement daily for four weeks, 76 of 82 patients reported significant decreases in pain as measured by the "Arhus low back pain rating scale."

Life on earth depends on appropriate pH levels in and around living organisms and cells. Human life requires a tightly controlled pH level in the serum of about 7.4 (a slightly alkaline range of 7.35 to 7.45) to survive.

Sickle Cell and Organic Food

I have been posting a lot about healthy living, good food that is favourable for someone with Sickle Cell. One thing that I have tried to do is – to buy organic food. The fresher the food, the better for us. Genetically modified foods are not good for the human body.

On the www.soilassociation.org website, it says:

Whatever you're buying – from cotton buds to carrots – when you choose organic, you choose products that promote a better world.

Organic means higher levels of animal welfare, lower levels of pesticides, no manufactured herbicides or artificial fertilisers and more environmentally sustainable management of the land and natural environment – this means more wildlife!

Going organic is easier than you'd think. Food, health, beauty and textile products that hold the Soil Association organic symbol have been produced to the highest possible animal welfare and environmental standards. Look for the logo!

When I was much younger, I could not care less about all this. I ate as much takeaways as I wanted and all. But now, with God preserving my life to this age, I owe it to myself to look after myself in a much careful and better way and do things the right way, whatever that is.

Sickle Cell and Food Rich in Iron

People with Sickle Cell tend to have iron deficiency. I have tried to compile a list of food that is good for us to eat and fight Sickle Cell and stay healthy and most importantly stay out of hospital.

Iron-Filled Food

Red lean meat, chicken liver, egg yolks, lentils, chickpeas, prunes, seeds (sunflower, sesame), Vitamin C, red peppers, broccoli, kale, berries, sardines in a can, boiled eggs, dried figs, spinach, beef, tuna, nuts (cashews, almonds, walnuts etc.), kidney beans, dried apricots, corn beef, dates, black eyed beans, shrimps, turkey, chicken, pork, oysters, lamb, cabbage, steak, raisins, bran whole wheat, sourdough bread, gammon, watercress, okra, veal, hot dogs, clams, peas, artichoke, potato (sweet or ordinary, with or without skin), pasta, pumpkins, pasta, lentils, spirulina, tomato (puree, sauce) bagel, breakfast cereal, wheat, quinoa.

Drinks

Orange, carrot, apple, cheery, grape, cherry tomato, strawberry – all juices. Red wine, Guiness, V8 drink and pomegranate as a drink or a fruit.

The list is by no means exhaustive. The main thing is, if you are eating, do try and consider to eat from the list because these are food high in iron.

African Nutritious Food

Black Velvet Tamarind: Black velvet tamarind has anti-inflammatory properties: the fruit pulp contains abundant vitamin C which helps to fight against microbial infections. Tamarind is high in many nutrients. A single cup (120 grams) of the pulp contains: Magnesium: 28% of the RDI, Potassium: 22% of the RDI, Iron: 19% of the RDI, Calcium: 9% of the RDI, Phosphorus: 14% of the RDI, Vitamin B1 (thiamin): 34% of the RDI, Vitamin B2 (riboflavin): 11% of the RDI, Vitamin B3 (niacin): 12% of the RDI.

Trace amounts of vitamin C, vitamin K, vitamin B6 (pyridoxine), folate, vitamin B5 (pantothenic acid), copper and selenium are also found in black velvet tamarind.

Coconut: Coconuts are especially high in manganese which is essential for bone health and the metabolism of carbohydrates, proteins and cholesterol. It promotes healthy brain function; protein containing coconut milk aids the digestive system, and it boost skin health. Coconut water is a great electrolytic drink, rehydrating the body at a cellular level.

Garden Eggs: Garden egg is a good source of dietary fibre, as well as other minerals and vitamins, such as vitamins B, potassium, folate, manganese, magnesium, copper, niacin and other various secrete nutrients which helps in the development of humans.

They are a natural source of vitamin B1, such as thiamin, niacin, B6 that helps the body in the proper use of fat and protein. Garden eggs also contribute to the nervous system positively and they are rich in anti-oxidants.

Guava: Guava is one of the richest sources of vitamin C; it actually contains 4 times the vitamin C content in oranges. Guava is loaded with nutrients.

Guava is also rich in other antioxidants, and has been shown to have a number of great health benefits. Guava contains more than twice the recommended daily allowance of Vitamin C. In addition to its high Vitamin C content, guava is also packed with other nutrients, including: Iron, Calcium, Vitamin A and Potassium.

Hibiscus/Zobo: Hibiscus is rich in vitamin C, which will help boost your immune system, which is good for people with anemia; it is high in iron, a mineral that keeps the immune system balanced and helps the body to maintain red blood cells.

It keeps your liver healthy because of its antioxidant properties; helps calm anxiety or depression (living with pain, constantly, can make one depressed); improves digestion; helps with sleep; helps in the prevention of kidney stones.

Include drinking a glass or mug of this drink daily and this will help you stay hydrated and increase the amount of oxidants that you consume. Anti-oxidants are molecules that help fight compounds called free radicals, which cause damage to your cells. It aids digestion. It will keep our immune system healthy too.

Jute Leaves: Jute leaves are said to be a good source of beta-carotene, which is why it is used in medicines in most parts of Africa and the Middle East.

Jute leaves are said to contain iron, protein, Vitamin A, C, and E; thiamine, riboflavin, niacin, folate and dietary fibre. The leaves are also said to have anti-inflammatory properties.

Moringa: Moringa has many important vitamins and minerals. The leaves have 7 times more vitamin C than oranges and 15 times more potassium than bananas.

Moringa also contain calcium, protein, iron, and amino acids, which help your body heal and build muscle. Moringa is packed with anti-oxidants, which are substances that can protect cells from damage and may boost the immune system.

Okra: Okra is sometimes referred to as 'lady's finger', okra comes in 2 colours: red and green. Okra is also an excellent source of vitamin C and it packs many anti-oxidants that are beneficial to your health. Both varieties taste the same and the red one turns green when cooked.

They rich are in fibre and the mucous like content in the okra pods helps ease digested food and constipation conditions. The pods contains vitamin (A, B complex, C and K) as well as a high amount of anti-oxidants. The pods equally contain good minerals such as iron, calcium, magnesium and manganese.

Okra boast an interesting nutrient profile: Magnesium: 14% of the Daily Value (DV), Folate: 15% of the DV, Vitamin A: 14% of the DV, Vitamin C: 26% of the DV, Vitamin K: 26% of the DV, Vitamin B6: 14% of the DV.

Plantain: They contain more vitamins and minerals than potatoes. They are rich in fibre, vitamins A, C, B6 and the minerals magnesium and potassium.

Sweet Potato: Sweet potatoes are nutritious, high in fibre, very filling, and delicious. It's rich in an antioxidant called beta carotene, which is very effective at raising blood levels of vitamin A, It is also rich in vitamin C, E, B5, B6, potassium, manganese and protein.

They can be eaten boiled, baked, steamed, or fried. Sweet potatoes are usually orange but also found in other colors, such as white, red, pink, violet, yellow, and purple.

Tiger Nuts: Tiger nuts are rich in vitamins and nutrients namely: vitamins C and E, iron, Magnesium, Zinc, Potassium and Calcium. Tiger nuts are also a rich source of anti-oxidants, which are beneficial compounds that protect your body against aging.

Ugu: It is called Sokoyokoto in Yoruba, Ugu in Ibo, Kabewa in Hausa, Ikong-Ubong in Efik and Pumpkin leaves in English. It contains calcium, iron, potassium and manganese. It also provides a good amount of the following vitamins: A, C, B2 an E.

The vitamin contents present in this vegetable helps in maintaining healthy tissues, cells, membrane as well as maintaining the skin and treating the skin of wounds in the case of vitamin C.

Ugu is rich in powerful anti-oxidants that offer some immune system and anti-inflammatory benefits.

The presence of iron and other important minerals in it contributes in the boosting of blood in the body system and prevent anemia. Ugu also contains a good amount of calcium that the body needs for maintaining healthy bones and teeth and also keep the skeletal system in normal functioning conditions.

Ugu contains magnesium which plays a vital role in making the bone firm, and strong, as it helps the adequate absorption of calcium by the bones. It also plays the same function on the teeth, as adequate magnesium in the body helps in making the teeth stronger and firm. Ugu also has potassium as one of the minerals it contains which also help in maintaining the bone mineral density.

Yam: Yam is not only an excellent source of fibre but also it is also high in potassium and manganese, which are important for supporting bone health, growth, metabolism and heart function. These tubers also provide decent amounts of other micro-nutrients such as copper and vitamin C. Copper is vital for red blood cell production and iron absorption, while vitamin C is a strong anti-oxidant that can boost your immune system.

It can be eaten either roasted, fried or grilled or boiled. Nutritional value content: contains vitamins (A, C, D, E, K, B6, B12 and more).

Contains anti-oxidants, carbohydrates, minerals, such a (Calcium, Iron, Magnesium, Potassium, Zinc, Copper) etc. All these will help with the fight against Sickle Cell.

Individuals with SCD are often low in these vitamins and nutrients. These deficiencies cause a significant depreciation in blood-antioxidant status in these patients, and the resulting oxidative stress may precipitate vaso-occlusion–related acute chest syndrome.

The consumption of food rich in vitamin C helps the body develop immunity against infections, reduced episodes of colds and cough and lastly protects the body from harmful free radicals.

If you want to know what these food are called in your country or local area, use a Google Translate.

PART 4: SICKLE CELL AND COMPLICATIONS

Complications of sickle cell disease are numerous. Acute signs may include pain in the hands and feet, fever, serious bacterial infections due to splenic sequestration/infarction, priapism, chest pain, shortness of breath, fatigue, pallor, tachycardia, jaundice, and urinary symptoms.

Chronic complications include delayed growth/puberty, retinopathy, chronic lung and kidney disease, cardiovascular disease, avascular necrosis of the hips and shoulders, bone infarcts, and leg ulcers. I have tried to compile a list of the most common complications of SCD below.

Acute chest syndrome. Sickling in blood vessels of the lungs can deprive lungs of oxygen. This can damage lung tissue and cause chest pain, fever, and difficulty breathing. Acute chest syndrome is a medical emergency.

Acute pain crisis. Also known as sickle cell or vaso-occlusive crisis, this can happen without warning when sickle cells block blood flow. People describe this pain as sharp, intense, stabbing, or throbbing. Pain can strike almost anywhere in the body and in more than one spot at a time. Common areas affected by pain include the abdomen, chest, neck, back, or arms and legs. A crisis can be brought on by high altitudes, dehydration, illness, stress, or temperature changes. Often a person does not know what triggers the crisis.

Aplastic crisis: Occurs when bone marrow stops making new blood cells. It is caused by certain viral infections in people with hemolytic anemias, such as SCD.

Aplastic crisis is usually caused by a parvovirus B19 infection, also called fifth disease or slapped cheek syndrome.

Parvovirus B19 is a very common infection, but in SCD, it can cause the bone marrow to stop producing new red blood cells for a while, leading to severe anemia. Aplastic crisis most commonly occur in newborns and children who have SCD.

Adults who have SCD may also experience episodes of severe anemia, but these usually have other causes. Babies and newborns who have severe anemia may not want to eat and may seem very sluggish.

Bacterial infection. Patients should be treated immediately if they experience any signs of infection. Patients should also stay current with vaccinations, including annual flu vaccine and less frequent vaccination against pneumococcus and meningococcus.

Chronic pain. Chronic pain is common, but it can be difficult to describe, but it is usually different from crisis pain or the pain that results from organ damage.

Delayed growth and puberty. Children who have sickle cell disease may grow and develop more slowly than their peers because of anemia. They will reach full sexual maturity, but this may be delayed.

DVT and PE. Sickling of red cells can increase blood coagulation and induce an increased risk of blood clot in a deep vein (DVT), or in the lung (PE) if the blood clot moves from the deep veins.

People with SCD have a high chance of developing DVT or PE. DVT and PE can cause serious illness, disability and, in some cases, death.

Enlarged spleen. If sickle cells become trapped in the spleen, the organ becomes enlarged and painful.

Blood pooling in the spleen causes damage, and hemoglobin levels drop in the body. This can be life-threatening and should be treated immediately.

Eye problems. Sickle cell disease can injure blood vessels in the eye, most often in the retina. Blood vessels in the retina can overgrow, get blocked, or bleed. This can cause the retina to detach, which means it is lifted or pulled from its normal position. These problems can lead to vision loss.

Gallstones. When red blood cells break down, in a process called hemolysis, they release hemoglobin. Hemoglobin then gets broken down into a substance called bilirubin. Bilirubin can form stones, called gallstones that get stuck in the gallbladder. The gallbladder is a small sac-shaped organ beneath the liver that helps with digestion.

Hand and Foot. Swelling in the hands and feet usually is the first symptom of SCD. This swelling, often along with a fever, is caused by the sickle cells getting stuck in the blood vessels and blocking the flow of blood in and out of the hands and feet.

Heart problems, including coronary heart disease and pulmonary hypertension. Frequent blood transfusions may also cause heart damage from iron overload.

Infections. The spleen is important for protection against certain kinds of infections. If you have sickle cell disease, a damaged spleen raises the risk for certain infections, including chlamydia, haemophilus influenza, type B, sepsis, salmonella, and staphylococcus.

Jaundice. A yellow cast to the skin and eyes indicates jaundice. Sickle cells die more quickly than normal red blood cells and can overwhelm the liver's ability to filter them from the blood.

This can in turn lead to a build-up of bilirubin (a byproduct of the breakdown of red blood cells) in the blood. The excess bilirubin results in jaundice.

Joint problems. Sickling in the hip bones and, less commonly, the shoulder joints, knees, and ankles, can decrease oxygen flow and result in a condition called avascular or aseptic necrosis, which severely damages the joints. Symptoms include pain and problems with walking and joint movement. Over time, you may need pain medicines, surgery, or joint replacement.

Kidney problems. Sickle cell disease may cause the kidneys to have trouble making the urine as concentrated as it should be. This may lead to a need to urinate often and to bedwetting or uncontrolled urination during the night. This often starts in childhood.

Leg ulcers. Sickle cell ulcers are sores that usually start small and then get larger and larger. Some ulcers will heal quickly, but others may not heal and may last for long periods of time. Some ulcers come back after healing. People who have sickle cell disease usually do not get ulcers until after age 10.

Liver problems. Sickle cell intrahepatic cholestasis is an uncommon but severe type of liver damage that happens when sickled red cells block blood vessels in the liver. This blockage prevents enough oxygen from reaching liver tissue. These episodes are usually sudden and may happen more than once.

Children often recover, but some adults may have chronic problems that lead to liver failure. Frequent blood transfusions can lead to liver damage from iron overload.

Osteomyelitis. Osteomyelitis (both acute and chronic) is one of the most common infectious complications in people with sickle cell disease.

Osteomyelitis is an infection in a bone. Infections can reach a bone by traveling through the bloodstream or spreading from nearby tissue.

Pregnancy problems. Pregnancy can increase the risk for high blood pressure and blood clots in women who have sickle cell disease. The condition also increases the risk of miscarriage, premature birth, and low birth weight babies.

Priapism. Priapism is an unwanted, sometimes prolonged, painful erection. This happens when blood flow out of the erect penis is blocked by sickled cells. Over time, priapism can cause permanent damage to the penis and lead to impotence. Priapism that lasts for more than 4 hours is a medical emergency.

Severe anemia. People who have sickle cell disease usually have mild to moderate anemia. At times, however, they can have severe anemia, which is life-threatening.

Stroke or silent brain injury. Silent brain injury, also called silent stroke, is damage to the brain without showing outward signs of stroke. This injury is common and can be detected on magnetic resonance imaging (MRI) scans. Silent brain injury can lead to difficulty in learning, making decisions, or holding down a job.

Other Possible Complications

Damage to body organs (like the liver, heart, or kidneys), tissues, or bones because of not enough blood flowing to the affected area(s). Sickle cells can block blood flow through blood vessels immediately deprive the affected organ of blood and oxygen.

In sickle cell anemia, blood is also chronically low on oxygen. Chronic deprivation of oxygen-rich blood can damage nerves and organs in your body, including your kidneys, liver, heart, tissues or bones and spleen. Organ damage can be fatal.

Orthopedic complications of sickle cell disease (SCD) include vaso-occlusive bone pain, osteonecrosis, and infections (osteomyelitis and septic arthritis). Individuals with SCD are functionally asplenic and are at risk for infections that may be life-threatening, and other bone and joint complications can cause severe pain and immobility that significantly interfere with functioning and quality of life.

Psychosocial complications: People with SCD suffer from a high incidence of social and behavioral health complications. Anxiety and depression have been reported to be as high as 28%.

Being constantly sick, may cause young children to miss school, limit college and job opportunities for young adults, and reduce career opportunities for older adults.

Such losses present significant financial challenges, often limiting access to health care, insurance, and necessary medications amongst other things.

Other issues that may affect patients' ability to manage SCD effectively, include navigating the time and transportation challenges involved in seeing numerous health care specialists while trying to work and take care of family responsibilities.

It is not uncommon for patients to see ophthalmologist, orthopedic surgeon, nephrologist in addition to a Sickle cell specialist (hematologist) and their primary care team.

A very rare form of kidney cancer (renal medullary carcinoma) has been associated with sickle cell trait. It is a rare cancer of the kidney.

Part 5: OTHER ISSUES AFFECTING PEOPLE LIVING WITH SICKLE CELL

Sickle Cell: Rejection and Coping Strategies

Rejection is an almost unavoidable aspect of being human. No one has ever succeeded in love or in life without first facing rejection and the same is for people living with Sickle Cell. We have all experience it, and yet, those times when we do are often the times we feel the most alone, outcast, and unwanted.

In fact, so much of the hurt and struggle we endure isn't just based on the pain itself but on what we tell ourselves about the experience, the cruel ways we put ourselves down or flood ourselves with hopeless thoughts about the future. Studies even show that our reaction to rejection is also based on elements and events from our past, like our attachment history. As a result, how we react to rejection is often equally or even more significant than the rejection itself. This is why learning how to deal with rejection is so important!

There are many ways to learn to deal with rejection. These include psychological tools and techniques that involve reflecting on our past, enhancing our self-understanding, and strengthening our sense of self in order to feel stronger in coping with current struggles and facing the future.

Here we highlight some of the most powerful personal strategies for how to deal with rejection.

Coping Strategies

Research suggests that self-regulation, which involves monitoring and controlling one's emotional and behavioural responses, may be the key to coping with rejection sensitivity. For instance, when you perceive a potential sign of rejection, it may help to stop and reflect on the situation rather than responding immediately. One way to do this is to look for alternative explanations for the behaviour instead of assuming the worst. If you're unable to make these changes on your own, you may need to enlist the help of a counsellor.

It can be scary to take steps to grow closer to someone because the deeper the relationship grows, the more the thought of being rejected could be. But learning how to build deeper, healthier connections is key to reducing loneliness and isolation.

Rejection sensitivity is not something you should ignore. In fact, symptoms often worsen over time if they're left untreated. Consequently, if you're prone to overwhelming emotional reactions including intense anger, anxiety, and sadness when you feel criticised or rejected, talk to a counsellor or a friend who knows how to listen well. Learning to address your sensitivity and respond more appropriately to rejection is the key to improving your overall quality of life.

Revive Your Self-Worth

When your self-esteem takes a hit it's important to remind yourself of what you have to offer (as opposed to listing your shortcomings). The best way to boost feelings of self-worth after a rejection is to affirm aspects of yourself you know are valuable.

Make a list of five qualities you have that are important or meaningful — things that make you a good relationship prospect (e.g., you are supportive or emotionally available), a good friend (e.g., you are loyal or a good listener), or a good employee (e.g., you are responsible or have a strong work ethic). Then choose one of them and write a quick paragraph (write, don't do it in your head) about why the quality matters to others, and how you would express it in the relevant situation. Applying emotional first aid in this way will boost your self-esteem, reduce your emotional pain and build your self-worth.

As social animals, we need to feel wanted and valued by the various social groups with which we are affiliated. Rejection destabilises our need to belong, leaving us feeling unsettled and socially unleashed. Therefore, we need to remind ourselves that we're appreciated and loved so we can feel more connected and grounded.

If your work colleagues didn't invite you to lunch, grab a drink with members of your church instead. If your kid gets rejected by a friend, make a plan for them to meet a different friend instead and as soon as possible. And when a first date doesn't return your texts, call your grandparents and remind yourself that your voice alone brings joy to others.

Self-love

Love is the very essence of life. It doesn't have to be earned, you don't have to wait for someone to give it to you, and you can never be found worthless of it. Love is never in short supply.

It is abundant, inexhaustible, easily accessed and free! Love yourself, you are lovable; get rid of your mental bad habits, and counter unhealthy beliefs with healthier ones.

Acceptance

Make a conscious effort to accept the vessel you were born into, not as a limiting factor in your life, but as an ally. When you come to accept the present circumstance as it is and appreciate that the past is behind you, you'll feel the power you have now, in this present moment, to consciously architect your future.

This in turn will help you stop judgements of right and wrong about your past, your parents, or who you are. This will equally help your acceptance of what is present in the here and now; as you stop the blame game. You have your life ahead of you, what do you want your legacy to be? How do you want your life to matter? How do you want to be remembered?

Rather than fighting your natural impulses because you fear what others will say or think about you, you'll learn to accept your desires as they are. Once you accept yourself, you become mindfully aware of your human tendencies and can heal your wounds and reclaim your perfection.

Accountability

Next, aim at thriving. It's up to us to create a life we love. Accountability shifts the ownership and stewardship of our life back to us. This can be terribly frightening and tremendously freeing. You are free to create a written description of '**the you**' that you desire or intend to be.

You may consider this your ideal self, if you like. This version of you may not be perfect or flawless, but this version of you lives an authentic life and is fully aligned with your personal values, motivations, and ideals.

Accountability is the process of taking personal responsibility for your life without guilt, shame or "pity parties" and move on to creating a life you'll love.

It may be scary to no longer assign blame on others, and recognise that your future is your total responsibility.

This may fill you with a heavy sense of dread, but know this, you can and will get past this fear. And soon you will re-experience the childlike wonder and joy of having a world of possibilities open to you.

Actions to counter rejection:

Affirmation: Use your words to build yourself up; positive self-talk, be your biggest cheerleader.

Service: Give yourself to help other when you can; service is a higher power.

Gifts: Invest in yourself; spend money on perfecting your crafts, education, training and vocation.

Touch: Don't suffer in silence, talk to people, an aunty/uncle, a friend a counsellor etc…

God: Whatever your belief system is, dig deeper into God.

Rejection is never easy but knowing how to limit the psychological damage it inflicts, and how to rebuild your self-esteem when it happens, will help you recover sooner and move on with confidence when it is time for your next date or social events.

Sickle Cell and Mental Health

Medical haematology teams all over the world, have been studying and looking deep into the issues of having a long term illness like Sickle Cell, constant chronic pains and its psychological impact on the patient. This research has been going on for a while but it is now coming to the forefront.

The management of sickle cell disorder (SCD) continues to pose a challenge to both haematologists and affected patients. Treatment advances over a generation have greatly improved the quality of life and longevity of patients. Nonetheless, the current position in terms of the identification of the clinical implications of psychological complications and management within a multidisciplinary context remains unsatisfactory. Haematologists have only begun to address this issue recently.

This review examines the evidence for some of the common psychological complications found across the life span of patients with sickle cell disease (SCD), which are likely to be encountered by haematologists responsible for their medical management. Electronic searches of medical and psychological databases were conducted with a focus on three main areas: psychological coping, quality of life and neuropsychology.

Psychological complications were identified in both children and adults with SCD, and included inappropriate pain coping strategies; reduced quality of life owing to restrictions in daily functioning, anxiety and depression; and neurocognitive impairment.

Psychological impact in patients with SCD mainly result from the impact of pain and symptoms on their daily lives and society's attitudes towards them.

Early research in psychological aspects of SCD examined the extent of its impact on both children and adults, and the functioning of affected families. These studies showed that the most frequent psychological problems encountered include increased anxiety, depression, social withdrawal, aggression, poor relationships and poor school performance.

A few case reports also indicated high levels of parental anxiety, overprotection, excessive feelings of responsibility and guilt. The psychological impact of SCD on individuals may be grouped into a set of illness-related tasks:

Adjusting to the symptoms and incapacities;

Maintaining adequate relationships with health professionals;

And managing the emotional and social consequences of the illness.

The extent to which individuals are affected by SCD may therefore be determined by their coping responses, as dealing with its continuous demands requires the acquisition of new skills and modifications to daily life.

The relationship between medication use and the pain experienced as a result of SCD seems to be complex, especially regarding opioid analgesia. For example, studies have shown that patients with SCD use more opioids as pain intensity increases.

Yet the concerns of some sickle cell patients who are over-treated with opioids in hospital, and the issue of dependency on opioids as a result of hospital treatment, have been documented.

It may be the case that health professionals have poorly understood pain and medication use in patients with SCD. Many doctors, including haematologists, have found it difficult to treat patients with severe pain who require frequent hospitalizations. These patients, sometimes referred to as 'problem patients', usually demand very high doses of opioids.

In addition, the notion that a considerable number of patients may be psychologically dependent on opioids is unfounded, and rather seems to be associated with other factors such as mood and activities, and inappropriate pain related behaviour or coping mechanism.

Sickle cell disease has profound effects on the physical health, as well as the psychosocial and emotional health of young patients. As with most chronic diseases, depression and other psychiatric disorders are common in SCD.

Rates of depression are similar to those found in other serious chronic medical disorders, ranging from 18% to 44%, and are increased over rates in the general population even when studied for illness-related physical symptoms.

In a Nigerian study, subjects with SCD had a prevalence rate of depression greater than those with cancer or malaria (but less than those with HIV/AIDS). While studies of depression in children with SCD have shown mixed results.

Children experience high rates of fatigue and other somatic complaints, impaired self-esteem, feelings of hopelessness in the context of frequent hospitalizations, absences from school, and the inability to experience a normal childhood. There are many potential contributing causes to symptoms of depression and anxiety in SCD. These include the chronicity of the illness; unpredictability of crises; chronic pain; overwhelming nature of medical complications, including anemia, fatigue, growth retardation, physical deformities, leg ulcers, renal failure, strokes and substantially reduced life expectancy; and racial prejudice and stereotyping. SCD may result in social derision, disability, and financial stress as well as stigmatization for pseudo-addiction to opioid analgesics.

One study found that adults with SCD had lower self-esteem than those with HIV/AIDS or cancer. Chronically prescribed opioids may likewise contribute to a component of substance-induced mood disorder.

Children with SCD are often underweight, shorter than normal children, and have delayed puberty; with their small stature, adolescents with SCD encounter problems with self-esteem, dissatisfaction with body image, and social isolation, with participation in athletics also limited due to fear of initiating a vaso-occlusive crisis. School performance suffers when hospitalizations lead to missing multiple school days. Accordingly, adolescents often experience hopelessness and social withdrawal.

PiSCES (a phase of research to describe medical trials) found that 27.6% of adults with SCD were depressed and 6.5% had anxiety disorder.

Depressed subjects had pain on significantly more days than non-depressed subjects (mean pain days=71.1% versus 49.6%, $P<.001$).

On non-crisis days, depressed subjects had higher mean pain, distress from pain, and interference from pain than those without depression. Both depressed and anxious subjects had poorer functioning on all dimensions of HRQOL (health related quality of life), even after controlling for demographics, hemoglobin type, and pain. The anxious subjects had more pain, distress from pain, and interference from pain, both on non-crisis days and on crisis days, and used opioids more often. Anxious patients were also more likely to be emergency room "frequent flyers."

Sickle Cell and Will Power

I had my quarterly haematology appointment and heard these two guys speaking in the waiting area. One might be in his late twenties and the other in his thirties. I enjoyed listening to what they were saying because in my social circle, I have no one who suffers from Sickle Cell that I can talk to or compare notes with about how Sickle Cell affects one's will to live.

Anyway, back to the the two young men, they were talking about not allowing Sickle Cell to stop them from fulfilling their destiny and purpose. I of course became quite interested in their conversation. Then one of them mentioned the power of 'willpower'.

The young men in the hospital were talking about not letting anything hold them back and not allowing someone say to them that something cannot be done and I thought, how interesting because, what they were talking about just described me. One said he would use willpower to not let a pain get to him, if he had something to do. Sound familiar?

I said to them that we are warriors, the guys next to me, who had his back turned to me turned around to look at me, as his friend whom he was speaking to and was facing me from afar, smiled.

As someone with Sickle Cell, I can say that we are warriors, striving on in the face of adversity and in the midst of pain. That is what I told the young men, as I felt, it was not nice listening in, relating to what they were talking about and not invite myself into the conversation. After all, they were not talking quietly and we were all in a public place.

I got nods of agreement from both of them like, yes, that is the word, after 'willpower', we are warriors and they said YES!

That word 'willpower' stayed with me, as I was called in to see my consultant and till I got home. I decided I would write about this as, anyone with Sickle Cell needs to have that fighting spirit within. The definition of willpower is – *control exerted to do something or restrain impulses.* Or it could mean – *determination, strength of will, strength of character, firmness of purpose, fixity of purpose, resolution, resolve, resoluteness, purposefulness, single-mindedness, drive, commitment, dedication, doggedness, tenacity, tenaciousness, staying power, backbone and spine* etc…

As I read all the synonyms of the word 'will power' from the internet, I recognised these words in me; I admit to being determined to get something done, when I was feeling unwell and no one knew.

I acknowledged the characteristic of commitment in the things that I do. I own up to how I have a 'staying power' to my detriment, when I should have cried for help and the list goes on. I am sure that you also recognise the above in yourself or in the life of your loved one with SCD.

This year and beyond, keep on looking after yourself as you keep on being resolute, purposeful and tenacious about your life, your work, your health, your desire to not fall sick and in your pursuit of happiness.

Sickle Cell and Depression

I want to talk about the issue of Sickle Cell and depression. Do people with Sickle Cell suffer from depression? I believe the answer is yes. As you know, when one is having a full blown Sickle Cell crisis, you become an invalid, unable to do anything for yourself and the pain is so much that one can barely speak.

Say for example you have a good job and you fall ill regularly; do you think your boss will be understanding? Some might but most won't. Whatever stage you are in life, being sick all the time will limit you and pull you back compared to your peers who have good health. Years ago, I had the head of my department tell me that he would not me as an executive. I bet you that one of the reasons why he said so, was because I took time off sick more than the others. I owed it to myself to prove him wrong and I did because I am now more than an executive, I am an author of books, a columnist, a blogger and my own boss lady.

I remember when I was little, my parents would always celebrate the birthdays of my siblings and mine. I would be the one to either fall ill the night before the birthday party or the evening of my party. So, as a child, I felt low that the party had to be cancelled because of me.

Or it could be a situation whereby I was getting ready to sit for an exam and again due to the stress of it all, on the day of the exam or during the exam, I am unable to sit for the exams because of SC vaso-occlusive crisis. Once again, this undermined my plan for the future.

When we were growing up, my siblings and I travelled overseas a lot due to my father's job as a career diplomat, an ambassador. Again, just before the day of travel, I would fall ill. Invariably over the years, I don't believe in booking my holidays in advance. I tend to book my tickets at short notice.

Again, there is this stigma attached to people with Sickle Cell and marriage, where the other partner would not want to settle down with someone who suffers from Sickle Cell. This is a shame, as if properly managed, the Sickle Cell sufferer can live a very happy, healthy and fulfilled life.

Ultimately, what I am saying is that Sickle Cell can make the patient suffer from melancholy, as it affects various areas of ones' life. The more often one is sick, the easier it is to become depressed.

What is the solution to depression in the life of someone with Sickle Cell?

Exercising helps as it increases serotonin and endorphins.

1. Eat well and healthily.

2. Get some counselling

3. Go to support groups.

4. Listen to music that you like, music helps lift up moods.

5. Listen to positive messages from people that you admire.

6. Try to manage your stress levels.

7. Look after yourself, so that you don't fall sick too often.

Sickle Cell and Health Fitness

What is health and fitness?

In order for you to be healthy, you will have to be fit and by that I mean getting in shape or having an exercise regime. I suppose it's about being mindful of your diet as well; by eating what is good for you as well as keeping fit. Not eating well will defeat the whole purpose of trying to keep fit.

Regular exercise improves health and fitness. Health is defined as a state of complete mental, physical and social well-being; not merely the absence of illness or infirmity. Fitness is the ability to meet the demands of the environment.

One of the links between physical activity and your health are, people who enjoy regular physical activity have lower death rates than people who have no risk factors but who aren't physically active. What's more, people who are physically fit live longer and have fewer heart attacks than patients who aren't physically fit. The facts are clear: Regular physical activity benefits people in general.

A regular physical activity program helps:

- Lower blood pressure.

- Increase HDL "good" cholesterol in your blood.

- Improve blood sugar.

- Reduce feelings of stress.

- Control body weight.

- Make you feel good about yourself.

The terms 'health' and 'fitness' are often used interchangeably these days, but there are important differences between them, even though they do interact. Let me explain.

'Health' is a general term describing the overall status of a person. Being 'in good health' implies being free from illness or disease, and not suffering from any impairment or pain. It's rather vague, but being healthy does not necessarily mean that you are fit. And health can be affected by many things – food, environment, disease etc.

'Fitness' on the other hand, is more a measure of the amount of physical capability than a measure of well-being. Fitness is almost entirely a result of action. Certainly food and drink can influence fitness. But the main way of increasing fitness is through exercise. And increasing your fitness has been shown to boost health is so many different ways:

Reduction in risk of cardiovascualr disease, reduction in the risk of contracting many cancers, and boosting the immune system being just three of them.

Personally, I love walking. For someone with Sickle Cell, eating well is very important. I mean food that is good for you and can help you minimise having a crisis and to have an exercise regime that is not too strenuous on you physically.

Sickle Cell and Addiction

Apparently anyone who suffers from SCD can be addicted to one or various pain killers, namely: pentazocine, naproxen, tramadol, diazepam, codeine and morphine etc.

This is quite serious and there is no simple solution to the matter. First of all, not all sickle cell sufferers are addicted to prescribed tablets. When someone has a crisis, he or she will most probably take one or more of the above, in order to ease the pain. When the pain eases, some sickle cell sufferer might want to keep on taking the tablets in order to continue to have that high feeling.

On a personal note, I use these tablets as a last resort because I hate the way they make me feel. When I use these strong opioids painkillers, I am unable to sleep and so it feels as if I am hallucinating and by that I mean I am in a place where it is difficult to describe my feelings while in pain.

Also, after taking these strong pain killers, I am left constipated, with stomach cramps and my stomach is bloated plus I then have to sleep a lot afterwards, in order to get the tablets out of my system and drink with plenty of water. All in all, not a positive post opioid experience and so I try to not take them till I really have to.

Medical personnel also assist in keeping SC patients stigmatised about being addicts to pain killers. Whenever I have had to go to hospital when having a crisis, I am treated with such contempt when I am asking for more pain killers. The situation really upsets me because I am sure that these people have no clue about the kind, type of pain that is ravaging my body.

How dare they, the nurses and doctors withhold any form of relief? In some cases, some people are in pain continuously and take these tablets in order to keep the pain at bay and it equally helps them to function normally on a day to day basis, especially, if that person has a job whereby they cannot afford to take time off work. As with anything in life, if you keep doing something over and over again, it will become a habit; albeit a good or bad one.

Now, how can a patient try and help himself or herself? How can someone who is dependent on drugs, come off it? Some people say taking other opiate replacements is the answer. My unsolicited advice would be to wean yourself off the medication, but it might be too much to stop all at once.

There is something that is very important before attempting to cut off addiction to any pain medication. And that is to have a very strong will that you will come off this addiction. You have to want to quit. You also have to stick to it. It is not an easy route because your mind will justify things to you and tell you, you need the tablets.

You might think to yourself that it would be okay if you just took the tablets once more today, because you will take one less tomorrow. When quitting pain medication it is very imperative to stick to the original plan. Deviating from that plan will more or less delay the process and make the withdrawal last longer. For those of you who are on high doses of pain medication, it may be necessary to wean down the amount that you take before quitting as going cold turkey can seem impossible. Most significantly, speak to your doctor about your dependency on pain killers.

Other things that can help are: Drink lots of water. Nothing better than to filter the body and help get rid of the junk in your body fast.

The more water the better! Teas without caffeine help. There is a tea called "Sleepy time" that really does wonders and will help you sleep as insomnia is a side effect of withdrawal. Caffeine is a stimulant and can increase withdrawal effects as well as dehydrate you. Vitamins and natural herbs help.

Anything you can do to give your body what it has been deprived from is a good thing. Watch out for herbs or vitamins that increase metabolism as the goal is to keep the body slow and slowly let it speed back up to working order. Nothing fizzy if you can help it.

Food has never tasted better after quitting pain medication. I've heard that fruits with lots of citrus are good. Another piece of advice would be to stay active. It is easy to want to sleep all day or sit in bed when quitting pain medication. While this can make the time pass I think it is better to stay active. Go to the gym or look for some exercises that are not too strenuous that your body can cope with.

During this time, you might feel depressed or lethargic and probably the best idea would be to do something that will take your mind off of the whole thing. It also helps to have people around you.

Sickle Cell and the Cold

I want to talk about Sickle Cell and the cold weather or being in an enclosed environment where it is cold.

As you know as a Sickle Cell sufferer, the cold is not good for us. Because when it gets cold, the red blood cells then clot together quicker and what happens next is a crisis. If you don't look after yourself when it is cold, the likelihood is that you might fall ill more frequently. When it is cold out there or inside, try and keep as warm as possible, by wearing layers, and if it becomes too warm for you, you can take a layer or two off.

I used to think the best way to keep warm is wear some heavy cardigan but the cold would penetrate through it quickly and before I knew what was going on, I would fall ill. I found out that it is better to layer up and by that I mean wear various layers of clothing this helps to protect oneself against the cold elements.

I have noticed that if I inadvertently expose myself to the cold weather, I would have a crisis, almost immediately. The same goes if I get caught in the rain, the consequences could be dire for me, with Sickle Cell.

If I unwittingly exposed myself to the cold, by the time I got home, I will feel the signs of something not right in my body. Nowadays, what I try to do right away, is to have **a very hot shower**, more like a sauna and after, I will eat and take my tablets and use a hot water bottle. So far so good, this personal regime has worked for me.

Dos:

Dress warmly but in layers and carry an extra pair of dry socks.

Stay hydrated (hot water, cocoa or herbal teas can be great).

Carry and use a hand sanitiser frequently.

Minimise continuous exposure to cold, windy or wet weather and snow.

Get plenty of rest and sleep, minimise stress, know your body and your limits.

Make sure you have pain medications handy to start early in the event of a pain crisis.

Don't:

Forget your hat, gloves and scarf when you step out.

Visit people who have a cold or febrile illness, if possible.

Drink too much coffee or caffeinated tea, since it can contribute to dehydration.

Get carried away with the ice skating, sledding or building a snowman.

Remember, being practical about guarding against the combination of cold and wet weather can go a long way in preventing a sickle cell crisis during the winter months.

Sickle Cell and Anger

If you suffer from Sickle Cell, then you will sometimes express impatience, be short fused, snap and also express emotions of anger. I have noticed, that I am more impatient during times of pain, and I don't necessarily mean being bed-bound. I shout and get short tempered or express emotions of anger easily. The pain is too much for me to bear and as such, the intensity of my expression of anger can also be heightened.

Of course, after my anger outburst, I feel remorse, as most probably, the person I was angry, impatient or even snapped at, was trying to help me.

Over the years, I have had to work on my anger and these guiding principles have helped me. In brief, they are:

- Anger is not evil
- Deep breaths before speaking
- Anger and stress affect our physical health (and our emotional, mental and spiritual wellbeing)
- Acceptance of personal responsibility and apologise
- Do you want to be right or happy?
- Personal commitment to not talk negatively if in pain
- Positive attitude, difficult I know
- Respect for the person helping me and acceptance of my situation

Look out for warning signs.

Sickle Cell and Oral Hygiene

The dental complications in sickle cell anaemia must be understood at first to efficiently treat SCD patients. Sickle cell disease (SCD) is one of the most common blood disorders typically inherited from one's parents. It is presented with a wide variety of clinical symptoms, and varied degrees of severity that can be determined based on the phase during which the disease is diagnosed, the age of the patient, number of hospitalisations in the past, requirement for continuous drug use and for blood transfusions, in addition to several other factors.

Acute infections can activate sickle cell crises. Therefore, it is imperative that dental infections should be prevented but, if there is an occurrence of infection, then effective ways of dealing with it should be devised immediately. A clear understanding of the dental implications of Sickle Cell Anemia (SCA), must be gained in order to successfully treat SCA patients. The treatment should always begin only after a thorough investigation on the patient's background has been performed.

The most frequent oral manifestations of SCD greatly affect the oral mucosa, gingival tissue, mandible, osteonecrosis, facial swelling, increased risks for caries nerve supply, and tooth enamel and pulp decay, basically tooth decay.

Dental caries are the most frequent dental complication worldwide. Patients with SCD are more susceptible to dental caries having more chances of tooth decay. Caries is identified as an infectious disease of teeth causing progressive demineralization and destruction of the enamel, dentin, and cementum of the teeth.

The key source of caries is the acidification of the oral environment, which is caused by the fermentation of remaining food particles mainly sugars or carbohydrates on tooth surfaces.

In addition, paleness of the oral mucosa, delayed tooth eruption, depapillation leading to atrophic alteration of the tongue, high degree of abnormality in the hypophosphatemic teeth, odontogenic infection, orofacial pain, craniofacial disorders such as protrusion of the midface area, maxillary expansion, mandibular retrusion, and maxillary protrusion. Dentists play a significant role in avoiding these complications and improving the quality of life in SCD patients as the SCD patients are more vulnerable to infections and periodontal disease.

Furthermore, these patients are at a higher risk of developing dental caries leading to elevated occurrence of dental opacities arising due to the unremitting use of medication containing sucrose owing to the high incidence of complications and hospitalization required by the lack of proper oral cleanliness.

Managing dental complications is frequently ignored as SCD patients are more dedicated towards maintaining a standard general health because of the serious blood disorder. Ignoring minor dental health matters under these conditions not only worsen the problem but can also cause a painful sickle-cell crisis, leading to emergency hospital admission.

Therefore, the management of oral complications in SCD patients require to be modified in accordance to their blood disorder, in order not to cause any additional deterioration to their overall health.

Sadly, the most commonly eaten diet these days is high in grains, sugars, and vegetable oils, and low in animal fats and fat soluble vitamins- the exact opposite of what doctors found to be helpful for optimal bone health and the prevention of tooth decay.

Nuts, for instance, have a high phytic acid content which can be greatly reduced by soaking the nuts in salt or lemon water overnight and then rinsing and dehydrating in the oven (the same can be done with beans). While this step is time consuming, it is feasible with things like nuts or beans, but much more intensive with wheat (which contains more phytic acid!)

Grains especially are better soaked, sprouted and fermented, if consumed at all, but this process does not completely eliminate the other harmful properties of grains. Avoiding the most common food sources of phytic acid can also help:

Diet to Help Heal Cavities and Improve Oral Health

1. Drastically cut foods that contained phytic acid. Limit the amount of nuts consumed; whatever what your daily consumption is, cut it to half.

2. Limited foods containing even natural sugars or starches– Limit fruit and even starchy vegetables like sweet potatoes and focused on mineral rich vegetables, bone broths, meats, and healthy fats.

3. Eat a lot of healthy fats.

4. Make an effort to consume a lot of homemade bone broth for its added minerals.

Other Helpful Factors

- Brush with homemade re-mineralizing toothpaste daily.

- I swish with both calcium and magnesium powders dissolved in water daily to help provide minerals and to keep the mouth alkaline.

- Some people brush with activated charcoal every couple of days to help pull toxins from the mouth.

- Also practice coconut oil pulling daily to help support tooth and gum health.

- Rinse your mouth with salt and warm water once or twice a day.

Sickle Cell and Walking

As someone with Sickle Cell, I grew up being pampered and well looked after and told I can't strain or stress myself and to be careful what I do.

What do we do with experts telling us it is important for everyone to exercise? Well, if they say it is, then it is, I guess.

I have taken up walking a lot, walking instead of taking the bus, or getting off three bus stops before or after my stop and walking. I don't jug, as when I do I become breathless and don't want to get back home and fall ill.

I try to walk from 30 mins to an hour at least a few days a week, when I can. Sometimes, I also carry my shopping as I go on my walk and that to me is as lifting weights. I sometimes power walk but walk leisurely mostly.

In the past, I also took up swimming as a pass time but the problem with that was the water getting into my hair and sometimes the water not warm enough for me. So I stopped.

Ultimately, you want to do something that you know your body can take, as you don't want to do something that will affect your body negatively, exercise wise.

What are the benefits of walking?

1. Walking strengthens your heart.

2. Walking lowers disease risk.

3. Walking helps you lose weight.

4. Walking tones up legs, bums and tums.

5. Walking boosts vitamin D.

6. Walking gives you energy.

7. Walking makes you happy.

8. Walking improves circulation.

9. Walking improves sleep.

10. Walking supports your joints.

11. Walking improves your breath.

12. Walking slows mental decline.

Sickle Cell and Stress

One major contributor to one having a Sickle Cell crisis is stress; let's look at the definition of stress and how we can manage it in our lives.

What is stress?

Stress is your body's response to certain situations. It's subjective, so something that is stressful for you may not be stressful for someone else. There are many different kinds of stress and not all of them are bad. Stress can help you act quickly in an emergency or help you meet a deadline.

Stress can affect your physical and mental health, and your behaviour. Your body responds to stress by producing chemicals and hormones to help you rise to the challenge. Your heart rate increases, your brain works faster, and you have a sudden burst of energy. This response is basic and natural. But too much stress can have harmful effects. It's impossible to completely eliminate bad stress from your life, but you can learn to avoid and manage it. Stress causes acidity in the body and increases free radicals – contributing to pain and inflammation.

Is all stress bad?

Not all stress is bad. In fact, some stress heightens your senses, helping you to avoid accidents, power through unexpected deadlines, or stay clear-minded in chaotic situations. This is the "fight-or-flight" response that your body triggers in times of duress.

But stress is meant to be temporary. Your body should return to a natural state after the situation has passed. Your heart rate should slow, your muscles should relax, and your breathing should return to normal.

The pressures and demands of modern life may put your body in a heightened state for a long period of time, making your heart pump hard and your blood vessels constrict for longer than your body can handle. Over time, these physiological demands can take a toll on your body.

Types of stress

1. Acute stress

Acute stress is the most common type of stress. It's your body's immediate reaction to a new challenge, event, or demand, and it triggers your fight-or-flight response. As the pressures of a near-miss automobile accident, an argument with a family member, or a costly mistake at work sink in, your body turns on this biological response.

Acute stress isn't always negative. It's also the experience you have when riding a roller coaster or having a person jump out at you in a haunted house. Isolated episodes of acute stress should not have any lingering health effects.

In fact, they might actually be healthy for you, as these stressful situations give your body and brain practice in developing the best response to future stressful situations.

Severe acute stress such as stress suffered as the victim of a crime or life-threatening situation can lead to mental health problems, such as post-traumatic stress disorder or acute stress disorder.

2. Episodic acute stress

When acute stress happens frequently, it's called episodic acute stress. People who always seem to be having a crisis tend to have episodic acute stress.

They are often short-tempered, irritable, and anxious. People who are "worry warts" or pessimistic or who tend to see the negative side of everything also tend to have episodic acute stress.

Negative health effects are persistent in people with episodic acute stress. It may be hard for people with this type of stress to change their lifestyle, as they accept stress as a part of life.

3. Chronic stress

If acute stress isn't resolved and begins to increase or lasts for long periods of time, it becomes chronic stress. This stress is constant and doesn't go away. It can stem from such things as:

Poverty – a dysfunctional family – an unhappy marriage – a bad job

Chronic stress can be detrimental to your health, as it can contribute to several serious diseases or health risks, such as:

Heart disease – cancer – lung disease – accidents – cirrhosis of the liver – suicide – Sickle Cell crisis

Managing stress

Stress affects each person differently. Some people may get headaches or stomachaches, while others may lose sleep or get depressed or angry. People under constant stress may also get sick a lot. Managing stress is important to staying healthy.

It's impossible to completely get rid of stress. The goal of stress management is to identify your stressors, which are the things that cause you the most problems or demand the most of your energy. In doing so, you can overcome the negative stress those things induce.

The Centers for Disease Control and Prevention Trusted Source recommend the following to help cope with stress:

- take care of yourself, by eating healthy, exercising, and getting plenty of sleep

- find support by talking to other people to get your problems off your chest

- connect socially, as it's easy to isolate yourself after a stressful event

- take a break from whatever is causing you stress

- avoid drugs and alcohol, which may seem to help with stress in the short term, but can actually cause more problems in the long term.

Outlook

Stress is a part of life and not all stress is bad. There are many types of stress, from minor incidents that last a little while, to chronic or long-term stress that is ongoing.

Stress affects everyone differently but it can lead to a variety of health issues. Managing stress is important to maintaining a healthy and fulfilling life.

Sickle Cell and Various Impact

SCD can impact on a youth's psychosocial well-being. Chronic illness can place significant stress on families emotionally, financially, and physically. Often communication and social support between family members and the hospitalised child or adolescent can suffer due to other obligations, time or financial constraints.

Chronically ill children often have a hard time with socialisation and adjusting to normal developmental transitions due to time spent in hospital and away from peers. Hospitalised and ill children and adolescents need social support and contact from family and peers in order to normalise and transition through development stages while also adapting to life with a chronic illness. Family involvement has been shown to produce better outcomes for the ill child, both emotionally and physically.

Many of the concerns with hospitalisation and social issues are common. Given that children and adolescents with SCD often suffer with feelings different than their peers, the desire to hide their disease to avoid judgement, and face social isolation due to frequent hospitalisations, better publicity of the social support network among SCD peers would be beneficial.

Aside from examining the idea of social support from other SCD peers, the support and communication with family and siblings is another issue. Four warriors in hospital were visited daily by a parent, for varying amounts of time based on age and parental obligations.

However, each warrior discussed missing their siblings often during hospitalisation and how much they enjoyed it when they were able to visit. The frequent hospitalisations can place a lot of stress on the family unit and disrupt typical social interactions between family members.

It has been shown that social support, especially from family, is a significant indicator of quality of life and adjustment for SCD children and adolescents.

Two of the adolescents discussed how they keep their illness a secret and do not want to involve their friends to avoid drawing unwanted attention or being viewed as different, a common fear among SCD children and adolescents.

Those frequently hospitalized warriors are removed from peers and social settings and missed their friends. The adolescent girl stated that she really enjoyed when she was able to speak with her friends and wished she could more often.

Both adolescents were still very dependent on their parents during a time when typical adolescents are seeking autonomy. The two children often missed out on physical activities at school and with friends due to hospitalisations and fear of painful crises.

The children described feelings of sadness and fear of getting sick, holding them back from participating in activities with other children. The children were not able to participate in physical education classes or sporting activities like their peers, reducing quality of life.

As noted above, recurrent painful crises represent the most common reason patients with SCD seek acute medical care. Painful crises most frequently involve the abdomen, chest, back, and extremities. Both the unpredictability and the severity of crisis pain contribute to its psychological morbidity and debilitation.

It is interesting that higher hematocrit is associated with more pain. Contrary to many studies of acute and chronic pain of other causes, men and women with SCD report generally similar pain experiences, both in terms of acute crisis pain and chronic pain.

PART 6: SICKLE CELL AND MEDICAL SCIENCE

- ◆ INTRAVENOUS IRON

- ◆ BLOOD EXCHANGE

- ◆ BLOOD TRANSFUSION

- ◆ BONE MARROW OR STEM CELL

- ◆ TRANSPLANTS

- ◆ GENE THERAPY

- ◆ HYDROXYUREA

- ◆ L-GLUTAMINE (Endari)

- ◆ VOXELOTOR

- ◆ CRIZANLIZUMAB (Adakveo)

Sickle Cell and Intravenous Iron

Iron deficiency I was told in hospital is when one's body can't produce enough of a substance in red blood cells that enables them to carry oxygen (hemoglobin). Iron deficiency leaves one tired and short of breath. One way of treating anemia is with intravenous iron, which is delivered into the vein, through a needle in order to increase the levels of iron and hemoglobin in the body.

Years ago, I went to the hospital for a routine check-up whereby I was told after a blood test that my iron level was very low. To be frank, I knew it, as I know my body and it gives me tell-tale signs. I had become very weak, to walk from a to b became a big deal, when in normal circumstances it's nothing. I had black circles under my eyes and any physical work I undertook, was draining on my physical body.

They booked an appointment for me to return to the Haematology day clinic in order to be given iron intravenously. Some people are given iron tablets and it works for them but unfortunately not for me, I react to it and so if my body needs iron, it will have to be given to me intravenously. Nowadays, I tend to eat a lot of vegetables, fruits and nuts rich in iron, in order to help me, so my iron level does not go down again.

For starters, I am one of those people whose veins are difficult to find. After six attempts from various nurses, someone is finally successful in putting the cannula in. Hurray, I said to myself, as I was fed up by this time and just wanted to get up, leave and say to them all, "I am not a guinea pig."

The sensation I was feeling inside of me as the drip of iron was going in was peculiar. It felt as if someone was slowly pouring ice like cold water inside of me. Halfway through the process, I was tangibly shaking and freezing.

When I get home, I still had chills and was feeling bitterly cold, even though it was not cold outside because it was summer. A previous time, after being given iron, I had a crisis because of this cold feeling on the inside.

After that incident of feeling frozen, I know what to do and know how to manage myself better: I go to the hospital warmly dressed in layers and I have noticed, that it helps me as my body temperature drops. I also took a flask of hot water with me and drank it all through and this helped me enormously. I also made sure that when I get home, I have a very hot shower or have a soak in the bathtub, as these steps help my body temperature to rise again and I take a hot beverage or soup. Lastly, I take some painkillers and then go to bed with plenty of covers over me or a duvet. It is strange how something that is supposed to help you, will now cause damage. I don't intend to have a crisis after being given intravenous iron ever again.

The last time I took all the above steps, I did not fall sick after being given intravenous iron. Now, I make sure that I eat food rich in iron on a daily basis so as not to be low in iron ever again. I'm growing and learning.

Iron is one of the minerals in the body. It is one of the components of hemoglobin, the substance in red blood cells that helps blood carry oxygen throughout the body. If you do not have enough iron, your body cannot make hemoglobin, and it may develop anemia.

SC and Blood Exchange

I was to have surgery and so my hematology team felt that it was important for me to have 'good' blood in me. The process was one of taking out my blood from one tube as another tube was feeding back into me the 'good' blood from the blood exchange machine.

Blood exchange was something that I had never had and I was intrigued about the whole process, and wanted to tell you all about my experience. I realise that some of you might have had blood exchange before or maybe your loved one who suffers from Sickle Cell, nonetheless, it is good to write about it for some other people who have not had it. Prior to my going for the blood exchange on the day in question, I previously had to go and have a blood test done, in order for them to ascertain my blood group.

On the day in question, I was told to get to the hospital for 9 am. I got there before the time said and the whole process began. It was a long day and I was very tired and in pain at the end of it all.

The bit that I found painful was them trying to get a vein in order to put the cannula tube in and as the nurse could not find any veins in my hands, it was decided that this whole process would be done through my groin and, was it painful! A femoral line, (this thing is bigger than a cannula tube) had to be inserted to my groin area.

I was also regularly monitored during the exchange (checking blood pressure, temperature, pulse and breathing rate) and asked how I was feeling.

Whilst there, I found out that some people have to come for a blood exchange every 4-12 weeks. Oh my goodness.

Let's educate ourselves on blood exchange for people with sickle cell:

An exchange blood transfusion – This is a procedure that replaces sickle blood with non-sickled blood.

Why would I need an exchange blood transfusion?

This procedure might be needed in an emergency, such as for:

• A complicated sickle cell crisis, such as a stroke

• A chest crisis – sickling in the lungs causing breathing problems

• A very painful crisis.

A routine or planned exchange transfusion may also be done in the following situations:

• If you have had a stroke, repeated exchange transfusions can help reduce the risk of further strokes happening.

• If your sickle cell disease is very severe, repeated exchange transfusions can help reduce the number of crises.

• In pregnancy an exchange transfusion may prevent complications to you and your baby.

• If you are going to have a major operation such as a hip replacement, a single exchange transfusion reduces the risk of complications from the general anaesthetic and surgery.

• If you have leg ulcers exchange transfusions may aid healing.

• An exchange transfusion may help in cases of severe priapism (painful erections) that have not responded to other forms of treatment or surgery.

What are the possible complications of blood transfusions?

Minor reactions – you may get a skin rash or a minor fever, for example. These can be treated easily with paracetamol and antihistamines.

Iron overload – This is common in people who receive repeated blood transfusions. When necessary, excess iron can be removed by taking medication (injections or tablets). This is much less likely when the exchange machine is used than when an exchange transfusion is performed manually.

Antibodies your blood is matched very closely with the blood of the donor (the person who donated the blood). However, it is possible to develop 'antibodies' against the donor blood. These antibodies can mean that matched blood is harder to find and can take longer to prepare.

Delayed transfusion reactions:

Occasionally a patient experiences a delayed transfusion reaction (where your body abnormally breaks down the blood you have been transfused), which may occur within the first two weeks of being transfused. This may cause:

• Severe generalised sickle cell pain/crisis

• Blood in the urine (red or cola colour)

• Feeling tired

• Feeling short of breath

- Fever

- Localised loin / back pain.

Having a femoral line inserted

A femoral line is a cannula (tube), which is inserted into the femoral vein near the groin to give one the donor blood. It is larger than a cannula for your arm. A femoral line is often needed to be used because the medical team need to use a large vein for an exchange blood transfusion, especially if the blood exchange machine is used. This is called an automated exchange transfusion.

You are given an injection of local anaesthetic to your groin, which is a medication used to numb the area so it is less painful. It takes about half an hour to prepare for the insertion of the femoral line, but it only takes fifteen minutes to put the line in. The line will need to be secured by a strong dressing or stitched in to stop it falling or being pulled out.

The femoral line is inserted by the advanced nurse practitioner or by one of the medical or specially trained nursing staff on the day unit at the hospital.

How long will the blood exchange transfusion take?

The exchange blood transfusion process can take from one to four hours on the machine. This will depend on your clinical history and how much blood will be used during the procedure.

However, you should expect to be in the day unit for the whole day (10am to 5pm). This is because the femoral insertion takes about 45 minutes and you should allow another hour and a half after the machine has stopped before you can leave the hospital.

What happens after the blood exchange transfusion?

When the exchange is finished, blood is taken from the femoral line so we can see how much of the sickle haemoglobin is left in your blood. The femoral line is then taken out and the nurse will apply pressure with their thumb to the area for about five minutes. You will be asked to lie flat for half an hour. This is to prevent bleeding. You will finally be assessed by a nurse and, if everything is fine, you will be able to go home.

Currently blood transfusion therapies increase the amount of iron in a person's body which can lead to serious problems such as liver disease or heart failure. Iron limiting therapy is required to reduce the amount of iron in the body, but this treatment can make some patients feel unwell and is very expensive.

Sickle Cell and Blood Transfusion

There are two kinds of blood transfusions:

They are very different: simple transfusions and exchange transfusions. Simple transfusions are used to deliver additional healthy red blood cells to the patient's body, while exchange transfusions exchange the patient's sickled-shaped blood cells with healthy ones, whereby lowering the concentration of sickle cells without increasing blood viscosity.

Simple blood transfusions are typically given in intervals, possible once or twice a month, to help maintain a healthy proportion of normal to sickle red blood cells.

Transfusions can also be divided into acute, long-term, and short-term transfusions. Acute transfusions are given briefly before surgery, short-term transfusions are given to assist a pregnancy, and long-term transfusions are given to prevent complications such as strokes.

When is a blood transfusion recommended?

Transfusions are either performed to increase the blood's oxygen-carrying capacity in case of severe anemia or to decrease the viscosity of the blood.

Transfusion to increase oxygen capacity

Certain situations make it crucial to increase the oxygen-carrying capacity of red blood cells in sickle cell patients. For example, an infection with parvovirus B19 can decrease erythropoiesis or the production of new red blood cells.

Since sickle red blood cells already have a reduced oxygen-binding capacity and are shorter-lived than normal red blood cells, such an infection can be very dangerous for these patients. In such cases, a red blood cell transfusion can be life-saving.

Sickle red blood cells can also become trapped in the blood vessels of the spleen, blocking blood flow, a complication known to occur in about 25 percent of sickle cell patients. This so-called sequestration crisis causes severe anemia and massive enlargement of the spleen, leading to abdominal pain. A blood transfusion is crucial in a sequestration crisis, helping trapped red blood cells to move back into the circulation.

Transfusion to lower blood viscosity

In patients with a high risk of stroke, blood transfusions may help to prevent stroke and brain damage. In such cases, transfusions need to be performed regularly. Anemia seen in sickle cell patients can also lead to acute chest syndrome (ACS), a condition where the oxygen concentration in the blood drops below a critical level, and breathing becomes difficult. ACS is a common cause of death in sickle cell disease patients and an exchange transfusion is strongly recommended within 48 hours of diagnosis.

Risks associated with blood transfusions

A patient who undergoes a blood transfusion may develop antibodies against the blood they receive, a phenomenon called <u>alloimmunization</u>.

This can cause serious complications, including hemolytic transfusion reaction, or a dangerous drop in hemoglobin levels to below those prior to the transfusion. To reduce the risk of alloimmunization, tests to match the blood group of the patient are used.

A blood transfusion can also lead to an excess of iron. This can damage the heart, liver, and other organs. Iron chelators, or medicines that bind iron, can help remove the excess iron from the patient's body.

Finally, blood transfusions carry a risk of infection but blood products that are used for transfusion are carefully screened, keeping the risk of infection low.

Sickle Cell and Bone Marrow Transplant (Stem Cell)

What is a bone marrow transplant?

Stem cell transplants (A stem cell transplant, also called a bone marrow transplant, is a procedure that infuses healthy cells, called stem cells, into the body to replace damaged or diseased bone marrow. Bone marrow is the center of the bone where blood cells are made) from bone marrow or blood of healthy donors are increasingly being used to successfully cure SCD.

In people with sickle cell disease, the bone marrow (the factory of the blood), makes red blood cells that contain haemoglobin S. This causes the problems associated with sickle cell disease. The goal of the transplant is to replace the cells that make haemoglobin S with cells that produce haemoglobin A.

Stem cell or bone marrow transplants are the only cure for sickle cell disease, but they're not done very often because of the significant risks involved. Bone marrow transplantations have been performed successfully in select children with sickle cell disease. Best results are obtained with matched sibling or related donors.

The next best option is fully matched but unrelated donors. Unfortunately, this second option is only rarely available. However, due to a lack of available donors and the risks of potential complications, bone marrow transplantations for sickle cell disease are not routinely performed.

163

- To prepare for a bone marrow transplant, strong medicines (chemotherapy) are given to the patient to weaken or destroy the patient's own bone marrow cells. This is done so that the patient does not reject the new blood cells coming from the donor.

- The patient is then given bone marrow from the donor who does not have sickle cell disease. The donor has normal haemoglobin or sickle cell trait. The transplant is given like a blood transfusion through an intravenous tube.

- The new bone marrow makes red blood cells that are healthy because they do not contain a lot of haemoglobin S.

Who can be a bone marrow donor? There are three types of donors:

- Matched related. A brother or a sister who has the same bone marrow type and the same mother and father who do not have sickle cell disease. Brothers and sisters are matched through a blood test called HLA typing.

- Matched unrelated. Volunteers who have the same bone marrow type as the patient. Unrelated donors are identified through national organisations.

- Haploidentical. Half-matched family members (usually a mother or father). This type of donation is considered experimental and is performed only as part of a research study.

Stem cells can be obtained from a donor's bone marrow or peripheral blood (blood in the veins). In some cases, stem cells are collected from the umbilical cord at the time of birth.

The cord blood can be stored for use in a brother or sister, or unrelated but matched cord blood can be obtained through a national or international cord blood registry.

What are the benefits of a bone marrow transplant?

Bone marrow transplant is the only treatment available today that can cure sickle cell disease. If the transplant is successful, the patient will be cured from sickle cell disease.

What are the possible risks of a bone marrow transplant?

Infections. Chemotherapy temporarily lowers the number of white blood cells, which normally fight and prevent infections.

• This puts the patient at high risk of infections which can be caused by bacteria, fungi or viruses.

• Medicines are given to prevent and fight these infections. However, some of these infections may not respond to the medications, although this is rare.

Graft-versus-host-disease (GVHD). This may happen when the immune cells of the donor sense that the patient's cells are different and attack them. This can be a serious side effect of the transplant.

- GVHD occurs in up to one in 10 patients who have transplants from related donors. It can be higher in transplants from other donors.

- This condition can be acute (occurring less than 100 days from the transplant) or chronic (occurring more than 100 days after the transplant.

- It may affect the skin, liver, lungs or intestinal tract of the patient.

- Medicines are given to prevent or treat GVHD. These drugs may increase the patient's risk of infection. However, the GVHD may not respond to these medicines and may lead to organ damage or even death although this is rare.

Graft failure. There is a one in twenty chance that the new bone marrow from the family member will fail to take. The chance of this is higher with other types of donors.

This means that the patient will not be able to make white cells, red cells or platelets. In this case the transplant will need to be repeated or stem cells collected from the patient prior to the transplant can be given back to the patient. This will restore the original bone marrow, which means that the sickle cell disease will come back.

Researchers are investigating new types of bone marrow transplants for children and adults with sickle cell disease. Several new approaches appear promising. They include giving less intense doses of chemotherapy prior to the transplant (a regimen known as "reduced-intensity conditioning"), or using low doses of immunosuppressive drugs or radiation in place of chemotherapy.

Nutrition problems. The stomach and intestines are sensitive to chemotherapy. Nausea, vomiting, mouth sores, diarrhea and loss of appetite may occur. The patient will be given nutrition through a nasal tube or through the veins until they are able to eat.

Low blood counts. The patient may require transfusions with platelets and red blood cells after receiving chemotherapy, while waiting for the new stem cells to make normal blood cells.

Infertility. Most patients who receive a transplant will not be able to have their own children in the future. This is a possible side effect of the chemotherapy, however there have been patients who were able to conceive children after having a transplant.

If the patient has gone through puberty before having a transplant it may be possible to collect and store sperm/ovarian tissue prior to the transplant.

Social and emotional concerns. A bone marrow transplant is challenging for the patient and the family members. The patient's routine will change for a while because they will be away from school, friends and relatives.

The average time spent in hospital is six weeks although some patients may have to be in hospital longer if they develop complications.

Who requires a transplant?

A bone marrow transplant is recommended for children and young people with sickle cell disease who have significant complications of their disease such as stroke, abnormal transcranial dopplars, and frequent vaso-occlusive crises despite the use of hydroxycarbamide. Two requirements must be met for the transplant to proceed.

- The first is to identify the best donor. This is done by blood tests.

- The second is to ensure that the patient and the donor are able to undergo the procedure. Both the donor and the patient have evaluations of the heart, kidneys, liver etc. In addition, interviews with a psychologist are important.

Is bone marrow transplant the only treatment for sickle cell disease?

Bone marrow transplant is the only cure for sickle cell disease at this time. Results of studies show that transplants from matched related donors offer a 90% (90 out of 100 patients) chance of cure. Other treatment choices are the drug hydroxycarbamide and red blood cell transfusions. These treatments lessen the complications of sickle cell disease but do not cure the disease.

Sickle Cell and Gene Therapy

Doctor Matthew Porteus remembers the first time he treated a patient in a sickle-cell crisis. The young woman was experiencing a deep, intense ache in one of her limbs. The pain, caused by a blocked blood vessel, is common in people with a blood disorder called sickle-cell disease.

Meeting that patient inspired Porteus to go into haematology, and to work on sickle-cell disease. Now he and other researchers want to rewrite the story for such patients, starting at the very beginning. They hope to cure sickle-cell disease while patients are still children, by editing the haemoglobin genes in stem cells taken from the children's blood-producing bone marrow, which can then be transplanted back.

The idea is that a single, albeit complex, treatment could spare children with sickle-cell disease a lifetime of missed days of school and work, hospital visits and organ damage. "To effect a long-term cure, we have to fix the stem cells," says Porteus, now a paediatric haematologist at Stanford University in California. Such a repair could potentially keep patients such as the one he encountered out of hospital.

To make the fix, researchers are turning to the gene-editing technique CRISPR. In the past year, several groups of researchers have altered haemoglobin-associated genes in haematopoietic stem cells — the precursors of all blood cells — from patients with sickle-cell disease, and a few groups have already transplanted the modified cells back into mice.

The lack of a cure for sickle-cell disease is especially frustrating for haematologists, because the condition is common and has been well understood for decades.

About 10% of people with sickle-cell disease are able to get a bone-marrow transplant from a healthy family member with a matching tissue type. However, the procedure is grueling: patients must undergo chemotherapy to eliminate their own bone marrow before the transplant. But in children, it cures the disease about 90% of the time.

If doctors could edit a patient's haemato-poietic stem cells — either to fix the β-globin mutation or to restart the production of fetal haemoglobin — and then use them to repopulate the bone marrow, there would be no need to find a compatible bone-marrow donor, and many more people might be cured.

"It's time we really concentrate on fixing this disease," says John Tisdale, a haematologist at the US National Heart, Lung, and Blood Institute in Bethesda, Maryland. "We have all the tools."

Part of the challenge, says Porteus, is introducing the guide DNA into the cell. If it is delivered as a naked molecule, by zapping the cell with an electric field that temporarily opens the cell membrane, then it doesn't last long. The cell senses it is being invaded and breaks down the 'foreign' DNA. To counter this, Porteus' research group is taking inspiration from gene therapy: they use a virus to deliver the repair guide in the form of a circle of DNA called a plasmid.

In November 2016, the team successfully used the viral approach to edit haematopoietic stem cells from patients with sickle-cell disease in the lab. "We can get genes corrected in 40–70% of the cells," says Porteus.

But after those cells are transplanted into mice with suppressed immune systems, their numbers fall off: 10% of the human cells that were incorporated, or engrafted, into the bone marrow of the mice produce healthy haemoglobin.

On the other side of the United States, two CRISPR-focused start-up companies are taking what they hope will be a less risky approach — interfering with genes that regulate fetal haemoglobin. CRISPR Therapeutics and Editas Medicine, both based in Cambridge, Massachusetts, hope to use gene editing to increase the production of fetal haemoglobin.

Unleashing fetal haemoglobin production is simpler than fixing the β-globin gene, because it doesn't require homology-directed repair. After the gene-editing enzyme makes its cut, the researchers' work is done.

The cell's DNA-repair machinery will take over, bringing the severed strand back together, and usually introducing errors that ensure the gene no longer works. This approach can be used to disrupt the function of repressors such as BCL11A, allowing edited cells to begin producing fetal haemoglobin.

Over the last 3 decades, several groups have worked toward achieving efficient and safe gene transfer to human chorionic somatommotropic hormone (HSC), HSCs for SCD as well as other genetic disorders. In order for gene therapy for SCD to become a reality, 2 main objectives must be achieved: (1) safe and efficient gene transfer or correction of long-term repopulating HSCs and (2) high-level, appropriately regulated, stable gene expression.

With current progress at the bench and in the clinic, these goals now appear within reach. The long path to the clinic for SCD gene therapies has been paved by landmark discoveries that have provided important insights into the developmental regulation of the β-globin gene cluster.

Gene therapy might one day provide a cure for sickle cell disease, but the technology is still in very early clinical and preclinical stages.

Nonetheless, there have also been advances in non-gene therapy treatment of sickle cell disease, such as better pain management, prophylactic transfusions, hydroxyurea, and continued research into experimental drugs like anti-sickling haemoglobin modifiers. Until gene therapy reaches fruition, these treatments represent the best opportunity for improved global management of sickle cell disease.

Why the caution? Children with SCD living in high-income countries no longer have a life-threatening disease, but rather a chronic disease with disease-associated, life-threatening events. Two large observational studies in children with SCD indicated 15-year and 16-year Kaplan-Meier survival estimates of approximately 99 percent with and without hydroxyurea therapy, respectively. A third cohort study of children with SCD from a region in Paris, France, indicated that after introduction of the online guidelines, there was also an increase in the overall five-year survival from 98.3 percent to 99.2 percent.

For children with SCD living in low and middle-income countries, where approximately 90 percent of all children with SCD are born, and gene therapy is not an option.

In summary, gene therapy to treat children with SCD is currently restricted to those who: 1) have severe disease; 2) have failed blood transfusion or hydroxyurea therapy; 3) require treatment for comorbidities; 4) live in a high-income country; and 5) are not likely to die from the disease in childhood.

Given the known short-and long-term toxicities of myeloablative (high intensity stem cell transplant) doses of Busulfan, the calculated trade-off of gene therapy is that the benefits will outweigh the unknown late potential adverse effects of Busulfan in this population.

Sickle Cell and Hydroxyurea

What is hydroxyurea?

Hydroxyurea is a medicine that can help children and adults with sickle cell disease. Research studies show that hydroxyurea lowers the following:

• The numbers of acute chest syndrome (pneumonia) events

• The number of pain crises

• The need for blood transfusions

• The number of trips to the hospital

Hydroxyurea also might prevent damage to the spleen, kidneys, lungs, and brain.

Hydroxyurea is given by mouth one (1) time each day. It comes in liquid or capsule form. The U.S. Food and Drug Administration (FDA) has approved it for the treatment of adults with severe sickle cell disease.

Which children should take hydroxyurea?

We consider hydroxyurea for children with sickle cell disease who have had:

• Many painful events,

• Several cases of acute chest syndrome (pneumonia),

• Severe anemia, or

• Other special problems with their internal organs.

How does hydroxyurea work?

Red blood cells contain hemoglobin. Hemoglobin helps red blood cells carry oxygen from the lungs to other parts of the body. People with normal hemoglobin have mostly Hemoglobin A in their red blood cells. People with sickle cell disease have mostly sickle or Hemoglobin S (Hb S) in their red blood cells. Hb S is an abnormal type of hemoglobin.

In people with sickle cell disease, Hb S causes the red blood cells to change from a round shape to a sickle or banana shape. Also, Hb S causes the red blood cells to become rigid and sticky. This leads to blockage of blood flow to important body organs, muscles, and tissues.

Hydroxyurea treatment helps the red blood cells stay round and flexible. This lets them travel more easily through tiny blood vessels. In part, this happens because hydroxyurea increases the amount of fetal hemoglobin (Hb F) in red blood cells. Newborn babies have Hb F when they are born. Hb F helps protect them from sickle cell complications (health problems) during the first few months of life.

With an increased amount of Hb F, red blood cells are less likely to change into the sickle or banana shape. In most people, the amount of Hb F decreases after the first few months of life. Some people have more Hb F than others. People with sickle cell disease who have higher levels of Hb F usually have fewer complications of the disease.

Is hydroxyurea a cure for sickle cell disease?

No. Hydroxyurea does not cure sickle cell disease. Hydroxyurea can greatly reduce some of the complications of the disease. It does not work if it is not taken as instructed. Usually, it takes several months before you will see results or get any benefit from the medicine.

It takes that long to reach the right dose of hydroxyurea. It is important to remember that hydroxyurea must be taken every day for it to work well.

Is hydroxyurea safe?

Hydroxyurea was first used as a treatment for cancer. It is a powerful medicine. But hydroxyurea is given at a much lower dose to children with sickle cell disease. No serious side effects have been seen in children with sickle cell disease. It does not cause hair loss, vomiting, weakness, or loss of appetite.

Many children with sickle cell disease have taken hydroxyurea for several years without problems. Hydroxyurea is very safe when given by medical specialists experienced in caring for patients with sickle cell disease.

In children with sickle cell disease it takes several months to reach the full dose of hydroxyurea. At full dose, the medicine should slightly reduce the number of blood cells in the body. One type of blood cell that can be reduced is a white blood cell called a neutrophil. Neutrophils help fight infection in the body. For this reason, monthly blood tests are needed to check the blood counts. If the white blood cells are low, the dose of hydroxyurea will be decreased.

The side effects of taking hydroxyurea for a long time are not completely known. In the past, there has been concern about a possible cancer risk while taking hydroxyurea. But, an increased risk of cancer has not been found in children and adults with sickle cell disease. Some of these patients have been treated with hydroxyurea for as long as 15 years. The risk of cancer appears to be no different for people who have sickle cell disease and are taking hydroxyurea than for those who are not taking hydroxyurea.

What tests are done to monitor hydroxyurea treatment?

Patients taking hydroxyurea usually have physical exams and have their blood counts checked every month. They will be seen more often if needed. If your child is part of a research study, then more tests may be performed. These tests help to determine the long-term risks and benefits of hydroxyurea for people with sickle cell disease. Areas of the body tested can include the blood, brain, kidneys, heart, and other internal organs.

Sickle Cell and L-Glutamine

And so, I went to an event organised by the Sickle Cell Society in London recently; it was about talks on clinical trials taking place for people with Sickle Cell. Medical science teams around the world are doing their utmost best to look for a cure and to that I thank them.

They are trying to advance science and knowledge about SCD in the 21st century. There are other tablets also in the clinical trial stages both in the US and UK.

I want to talk about L-glutamine therapy because it has been approved in US since 2017 for the treatment of Sickle Cell by the FDA (Food & drugs administration). Before a tablet can be on the market for general sale, the tablet would have gone through a lot of research stages before it gets to the clinical trial stage. Even then, it would have had various clinical trials in the guise of phase 1, phase 2 and phase 3.

Among patients treated with L-glutamine in the study, there were subjective reports of improvements in regards to chronic pain and energy levels. It was noted that those who took the tablets and have SC had fewer number of SC crises; fewer SC hospital admission and a lower incident of pain in general, over a period of 48 weeks, when the volunteers were being monitored.

In sickle cell disease, many of the complications and much of the suffering can be linked to the tendency of sickle red blood cells to stick to the endothelial cells that make up the inner lining of the blood vessels. This slows the travel of the red blood cells through capillaries, which often leads to blockages, or vaso-occlusion.

This blockage causes pain, inflammation and organ failure. In addition, sickle cell anemia patients may experience significantly reduced physical abilities.

L-glutamine has been shown to have another positive impact in sickle cell anemia patients by improving their exercise endurance. No major side effects were noted, nor were there any deaths or severe adverse events attributable to the L-glutamine treatment.

Sickle cell disease causes a great deal of suffering for millions of people. If you want to use L-Glutamine for yourself or your child, do consult with your medical doctor.

Sickle Cell and Voxelotor (Oxbryta)

Oxbryta (voxelotor) is an oral therapy developed by Global Blood Therapeutics to treat sickle cell disease.

The treatment is approved by the U.S. Food and Drug Administration for people with sickle cell disease, and had been granted fast track, orphan drug, rare pediatric disease, and breakthrough therapy designations.

Voxelotor is as an oral, once-daily therapy that is developed for treatment of SCD. It is designed to work by helping haemoglobin hold onto more oxygen as the red blood cells travel through the body. This keeps red blood cells in their normal shape and helps stop sickling.

As there is a desperate need for new treatments for SCD, voxelotor, if licensed, will offer a new treatment option for patients with SCD. In addition, voxelotor has been included in the priority medicines (PRIME) program of the European Medicines Agency, and granted orphan drug designation by the European Commission for the treatment of sickle cell disease.

How does Oxbryta work?

Voxelotor, the active ingredient in Oxbryta, is a small molecule that binds to hemoglobin and increases the protein's affinity for oxygen.

By helping hemoglobin stay in the oxygenated state, Oxbryta also inhibits hemoglobin polymerization and prevents red blood cells from becoming deformed.

This restores normal red blood cell function and oxygen delivery, reducing disease caused by the loss of red blood cells. It should also help reduce the risk of vaso-occlusive pain crises caused by sickle cells blocking small blood vessels.

Sickle Cell and Crizanlizumab (Adakveo)

Adakveo (crizanlizumab) is an anti-P-selectin antibody that was developed by Novartis and has been approved by the U.S. Food and Drug Administration (FDA) as a treatment for painful vaso-occlusive crisis events caused by sickle cell disease in patients 16 and older.

How does Adakveo work?

Adakveo contains a monoclonal antibody, a molecule made in the laboratory to bind P-selectin, a protein that is found on the surface of endothelial cells (the cells that line the inner walls of blood vessels) and in platelets (blood cells that are involved in clotting).

P-selectin normally works to control the flow of white blood cells through blood vessels and how they adhere to blood vessel walls during periods of inflammation and tissue repair, such as after an injury.

In sickle cell disease, P-selectin contributes to the adhesion of sickle red blood cells (cells with an abnormal crescent shape) to blood vessels, preventing blood flow through smaller vessels. This causes inflammation and vaso-occlusive pain crises.

By blocking or inhibiting P-selectin, Adakveo prevents this adhesion molecule from starting the process that leads to blood vessel occlusion, inflammation, and pain, and helps to maintain normal blood flow.

After two initial doses given two weeks apart in the first month, the treatment must then be administered once per month at 5 mg per kg of body weight by infusion into the bloodstream.

In patients with sickle cell disease, crizanlizumab therapy resulted in a significantly lower rate of sickle cell–related pain crises than placebo and was associated with a low incidence of adverse events

PART 7: SICKLE CELL AND OTHER RELATED ISSUES

- ♦ MORPHINE

- ♦ TREATMENT

- ♦ PERSONAL SELF-CARE

- ♦ SUPPORT SYSTEM

- ♦ PAIN MANAGEMENT

- ♦ GIVING BLOOD

- ♦ INSOMNIA

Sickle Cell and Morphine

Morphine is a strong painkiller. It is used to treat severe pain and, to treat long-standing pain when weaker painkillers no longer work. Morphine is only available on prescription. It comes as tablets, capsules, granules that you dissolve in water, a liquid to swallow, an injection or a suppository which is a medicine that you push gently into your rectum. Morphine injections are usually only done in hospital.

As someone who tries very hard to manage at home when having a crisis, before I finally end up in hospital, I heard someone saying in the outpatients clinic one day that 'sicklers' are drug addicts! I was like what?! No I'm not!

As I continued eavesdropping on the conversation, the dialogue was about how 'sicklers' like taking Morphine, street name Heroine, when in pain. As we all know, pain and sickle cell are good friends and pain embodies Sickle Cell. The two people (professional) I might add, were talking about the psychological dependence that people with Sickle Cell have with Morphine.

If you are a warrior, then you know that they say some of the tablets that we take can cause liver damage and other organ damage to the body. So for a while now, my principle has been to have food in my freezer, so that when I am sick and have to take very strong pain killers, I do so with food and I mean food health for Sickle Cell and not just take them with biscuits. This is my way of trying to make sure that as the tablets dissolves inside of me, it has food to help cushion it.

Some doctors do not like prescribing Morphine and they say, if you have to take Morphine at home, then you need to be in hospital, where you can be monitored.

The use of Morphine can be somewhat controversial amongst doctors. I have had some consultants not prescribe it for me and I have had some prescribe it. The thing is, I use tablets wisely, as I don't like to use tablets in the first place. I have been prescribed a box of Morphine and it expired in my tablets container with three quarters of it still left!

Yes, they say people with Sickle Cell go into hospital with chronic or severe pain and leave the hospital drugged up. Now this is true because whenever I am admitted into hospital, I usually spend a week there and I need another week off, in order to recover at home from the onslaught of all the morphine in my system. They say that people with Sickle Cell die from using opiates such as Morphine. They say morphine affects the brain negatively and also one's whole internal system.

Truth is, I am scared of using morphine at home when no one is with me, as I feel it's too risky but when I have a crisis and the pain is unmanageable, I would take it as a last resort. I have a fear of Morphine and steer clear of it till I have no choice.

I always say, thank goodness for science because they are always improving things. Now, I am prescribed slow-release morphine tablets and they work better in my system. I do still have the effects of normal morphine which are being bloated, constipated and vomit but I don't feel as drugged or spaced out as before.

When in hospital though, the protocol is to administer the injection every four hours however when the pain is unbearable, I might ask for it at three hours.

When I leave the hospital, it's true, I am totally drugged up and I sometimes need about seven days to get the after effect of morphine out of my system. So, be careful if you are taking morphine.

Key facts:

Morphine works by blocking pain signals from travelling along the nerves to the brain.

The most common side effects of morphine are constipation, feeling sick and sleepiness.

Different types of morphine

Morphine comes as:

Tablets (fast-acting) – these contain 10 mg, 20 mg or 50 mg of morphine.

Tablets (slow-acting) – these contain 5mg, 10 mg, 15mg, 30mg, 60mg, 100mg or 200mg.

Capsules (slow-acting) – these contain 10 mg, 30 mg, 60 mg, 90 mg, 120 mg, 150 mg, 200mg of morphine.

Granules (that you mix in water to make a drink) – these ae sachets containing 30mg, 60mg, 100mg or 200mg of morphine.

A liquid that you swallow – this contains 10mg of morphine in a 5ml spoonful of 20mg of morphine in 1ml of liquid.

Suppositories – these contain 10mg of morphine; useful if you cannot swallow tablets or liquids.

Injection (usually given in hospital).

Sickle Cell and Self-Treatment

The topic about self-management is very important in the life of someone with SCD. Over the years, people have asked me what I do to stay healthy. I decided to write something about it because if you don't make it a point of duty to know yourself and also to know how to manage this life-long disorder, then it is possible that one would be depressed all the time, one would have loss of appetite, not want to socialise or go out and feel lethargic continually. As a result, the issue of self-treatment is important.

I went to the user group meeting of the hospital I attend a while back and the focus was on self-management. If you have or are looking after someone who has SCD, then, it is important that you know or help the patient with SCD know about self-treatment, as it is a vital aspect of managing this chronic disorder. SCD is varied in the way it affects one person to the next. The key issues of self-treatment are what to eat, drink and tablets to take on a daily basis. They include:

Treatment of infections:

- Management of chronic complications as a result of Sickle Cell;

- What to take when you can feel the pain coming up;

- What to eat when not well;

- Knowing when to go to hospital as a day patient or go to be admitted;

- Prevention of complications in the life of someone with Sickle Cell.

For sickle cell crisis, when the severity of the episode is manageable, self-treatment can be sought at home with bed rest, oral analgesia, and hydration is possible and also recommended. I for one will present to the emergency department (ED) after self-treatment fails at home

PAIN – Vaso-occlusive pain episodes experienced by patients with sickle cell disease vary tremendously in frequency and severity. Some patients rarely have painful crises, while others spend the greater part of a given year in the hospital receiving analgesics.

The mode of onset of sickle cell pain crises likewise varies. Patients can develop agonizingly severe pain in as little as 15 minutes. In other instances, the pain gradually escalates over hours or even days. Patients manage most episodes of pain at home, until one gets to a point where all the medication one is use are no longer working.

Oral analgesics, combined with rest and fluids often allows the patient to "ride out" the pain episode. Some patients' report that warm baths or warm hot water bottles applied to aching joints ameliorates the severity of the pain. The sites affected in acute painful crises vary for each patient.

Pain occurs commonly in the extremities, thorax, abdomen, joints, chest and back. Pain tends to recur at the same site for a particular person. For each person, the quality of the crisis pain is usually similar from one crisis to another.

OPIOD -The pain experienced with an acute painful crisis typically is quite severe. Most patients describe a full blown crisis as the most intense pain that they have ever experienced.

The pain sometimes increases in severity slowly over a couple of days. At other times, a crescendo is reached in less than 15 minutes. Pain control often requires large quantities of opioid analgesics. The exact amount varies, and depends in part on the frequency with which the person requires opioids and how bad the pain is.

Patients often feel that one analgesic controls pain more effectively than others. Therefore, they should be questioned about the kind of medication that has worked best in the past. Also, some patients may experience reactions with one analgesic (e.g., itching with meperidine) but not with others.

Pain relief occurs more slowly with intramuscular injections, and the injections themselves can produce substantial discomfort. Consequently, intravenous administration of analgesics is usually preferable. As pain control improves, the analgesia should be maintained to prevent the patient from slipping back into a painful cycle.

Patients can become drowsy as their pain is controlled. Often, this reflects the fatigue that comes with several sleepless nights with pain at home. The analgesics should not be discontinued automatically as long as the patient is easily aroused. A common misconception is that if a person is sleeping, the analgesics are controlling the pain. Some patients often sleep despite severe pain and some don't sleep for days. The quantity of analgesia can be slowly reduced as the patient's symptoms improves. While the tapering of intravenous analgesics can require only two or three days, control of a full blown crisis often requires 10 to 14 days. Less commonly, bouts of sickle vaso-occlusive pain require several weeks to control.

NSAIDs can impair kidney function and accelerate the renal injury produced by sickle cell disease itself. For these reasons, many specialists avoid NSAIDs in patients with sickle cell disease.

TRANSFUSION – Simple transfusion is not an effective intervention for the management of acute painful episodes in patients with sickle cell disease.

Exchange transfusion has been used in attempts to alleviate bouts of severe, intractable pain with better effect, overall. In addition, chronic transfusion therapy has been used to decrease the frequency of pain in patients with recurrent debilitating painful crises. While sometimes effective, this approach as a number of problems, as detailed below.

Indications for urgent referral to hospital in sickle cell disease crisis:

- Severe pain not controlled by simple analgesia or low dose opioids

- Dehydration caused by severe vomiting or diarrhea

- Severe sepsis: temperature >38.5°C or >38°C if under 2 years old, temperature <36°C, or hypotension

- Symptoms or signs of acute chest syndrome including tachypnoea, oxygen saturation more than 5% below steady state, signs of lung consolidation

- New neurological symptoms or signs

- Symptoms or signs of acute fall in hemoglobin

- Acute enlargement of spleen or liver over 24 hours, particularly in young children

- Marked increase in jaundice

- Hematuria

- Fulminant priapism lasting more than two hours or worsening of recurrent episodes

- Acute infection

Sickle Cell and Personal Self-Care

As I write weekly as a columnist, I always have people getting in touch with me, wanting to know what I do when it comes to looking after myself. Well here is what I do, in order to look after myself.

I use a wide range of things, when in pain: hot water bottle/s, menthol creams, Ibuprofen cream, Pain patches, pain tablets (but I make sure I also eat something nutritious). I take anti-sickness tablets, try to rest, take very hot showers, use the electric blanket all night if need be, try to avoid stress as much as I can (easier said than done). We all know that when one is sick, the last thing on your mind is food, however, I cannot take all these strong painkillers like Morphine or Codeine, Diclofenac/Voltarol or Co-codamol etc… on an empty stomach.

You all know, I talk a lot about food in my blog, I try to eat a lot of green leafy greens like spinach, Ugu, Okra, Ewedu (Corchorus). I eat chicken, lamb or goat meat, (instead of beef), liver, kidney, tripe and fish. I eat all kinds of beans dishes. I eat other vegetables like corn, carrots and so tend to cook a lot of stir-frys (as I would then have an array of vegetables in it).

I start taking things like Ibuprofen or Paracetamol if I can sense that my body is not right. I try to keep warm, I drink plenty of water on its own or with lemon or lime (in order for it to be alkalised – it helps to neutralise acid in the blood stream) or ginger tea.

I take green tea (first thing in the morning because of its anti-oxidant properties). I make sure that I would have a full spoon of molasses with hot water daily, at night (molasses – lowest sugar content of any sugar cane product and has a lot of nutritional value).

If I want to snack, I would eat nuts or popcorn. And if biscuits, it might be digestives. I also feast on fruits that I like. Some fruits like banana or apples unsettle my stomach but they are good for you as an individual. I tend to eat more citrusy fruits, grapefruit, oranges, tangerines, and all manner of berries; I like fruits that have a bit of sweet and sour after taste.

I do try and eat well even though it can be quite difficult because I suffer from IBS and my belief is all the strong pain killers that I have taken over the years, have not done my stomach any favours. Also in the past, I tend to throw up quite a lot; thank goodness, it is not as much now. I think the anti-sickness tablets that I was prescribed did not go down well back then.

So, when it comes to food, I am choosy and fussy. I tend to stick to food that does not do me any harm, in terms of its after effects on me after eating. Also, I know that if I get caught in the rain, I will be sick when I go to bed that night, so I will take tablets beforehand. Or I now know if I am caught in the cold or the wind or if I am stressed out, I could be sick. I am at an age, where I know my body's triggers.

I have not hidden the fact that God is a strong part of my life and I would not be alive, doing what I am doing without His grace, favour and mercy upon me. I have verses of Scriptures from the Bible that I would repeat daily for a long period of time on healing.

Sickle Cell and Support System

As someone with Sickle Cell, I need a lot of care and rely on friends and family to support me when I am down having a crisis.

I have come to realise that what someone with Sickle Cell needs in their lives amongst other things is a close support network of people. Due to the unpredictable nature of Sickle Cell Anemia, one can be sick at any time and it is key to have people around you or have people that you can call on at very short notice.

I also know that people who suffer from Sickle Cell can be proud and not ask for help when it is needed. Please don't suffer on your own, in pain, when you can ask someone for a helping hand. I am fortunate to have a close network of friends and family, who would drop what they are doing at the drop of a hat, in order to come to my aid in my time of distress with Sickle Cell.

In order to receive help or get help when you are having a crisis, then on your good days, you also need to lend a helping hand to someone else. They say 'in order to receive, you must give'. This is so true, I cannot just be taking from loved ones' and not give something back in return when I am well an able to.

One should not sit around and say 'woe is me, I have Sickle Cell', I have nothing to give and I need help. No, look within, there might be someone around you that you too can lend a helping hand to. In order to receive love, you too must show love.

Sometimes, we can get self-absorbed with our issues and think, we are the only ones' suffering. The people in your circle of support could also be suffering from watching you unwell.

However, that is not the case, other people too are going through various challenges, and it is called 'life'. I want to encourage us to go out of our way to help other people. When I say this, I am not just talking about the ones' who are helping you. Of course, you will need to show your appreciation, gratitude and also love to those who look after you or take care of you when you were sick.

People who go through pain can sometimes be grumpy and short tempered; I believe it's because of the excruciating pain that we go through. Action they say speaks louder than words; if my people can come to my aid at very short notice when I am unwell, then I should be able to equally let them know how much I value what they have done or are doing for me, when the occasion presents itself.

Life does throw us curve balls from time to time; so there will come an opportunity where you too can be there for your friend or family member/s who helped you through your difficult times. I try to do what I can, in terms of helping my people and others when I am able to do so.

Of course, life can be hard, because of Sickle Cell, one could go to bed happy and stress free and wake up in the middle of the night with pains. Nevertheless, have you paused to say 'thank you' to those who have and are still helping you along the way? I am telling you this because when I am sick, I can lose patience quicker than normal and snap at a loved one. I therefore make a conscious effort to repay the love extended to me when I am able to do so.

Showing gratitude comes in so many ways: it could be in the form of a gift or giving your time; the point is do not just receive without making an attempt to also give back. You can also be there for your friend or family member, as they were there for you.

Sickle Cell is a lifelong sickness that will stay with one for life; except if you get healed supernaturally or go for one surgery or the other, available for people with Sickle Cell.

Bearing that in mind, it would therefore be a nice thing for you to also be a blessing in someone else's life when you see a need. I am hereby urging you to be kinder or more generous by being aware of how you sometimes come across towards your loved ones'.

Sickle Cell and Barriers to Giving Blood by Black People

Not too long ago, I was listening to the BBC London news, when they did a segment on Sickle cell disease and the lack of black blood donors. The report was an interesting one, as they highlighted the story of a young lady who has to have blood transfusion every six weeks.

The reason why this report was aired was to encourage the ethnic minority community to give blood because it is important for people from ethnic minority to give blood, so that this lady and thousands of others for example can be given blood from the right blood match.

The report said that there had been an increase in black donors in the last year however, 40,000 more donors was needed. A black blood scientist also talked about donating blood and said that the black community needs to step up. Apparently, some people in the black community are reluctant to give blood because they say that they don't know where their blood will end and they wonder if it will actually get to another black person.

However, another man who was interviewed said, when he gives blood, he gets a text telling him where his blood donation had gone to and he knows that it was another black person who desperately needs that well matched blood donation.

After listening to the short segment, I decided to do some research online about barriers among us blacks to giving blood and trust Google, there were write-ups about it. It is time for us to educate ourselves:

Minority blood donations have historically been low all over the world. Increasing the proportion of minority blood donations is essential to reducing blood transfusion complications, particularly in individuals with sickle cell disease (SCD) and thalassemia, for several reasons.

SCD and thalassemia disproportionately affect minority racial and ethnic populations. Individuals with hemoglobin disorders often need transfusions—sometimes habitually and sometimes intermittently.

If exposed to unmatched donor blood, the risk is alloimmunization: the development of antibodies to the foreign red blood cell antigens. Increasing blood donations among minorities can ensure better access to minor antigen-matched units; however, strategies for promoting donation in these populations require awareness of the unique characteristics of minority groups and blood donation, as well as programs that address facilitators and barriers to minority blood donation

Blood transfusions increase hemoglobin levels, increase blood flow, improve oxygen delivery to the tissues, and dilute the abnormal red blood cells containing sickled hemoglobin, thus increasing the number of circulating normal red blood cells.

Phenotypic incompatibility in blood transfusions results in the development of antibodies over time that attack red blood cells, making subsequent transfusions less effective and increasing the risk of transfusion complications.

The principal barriers to blood donation are inconvenience, perceived medical disqualification, being too busy, not being asked, and apathy. African Americans more often than whites cited bad treatment and poor staff skills as reasons not to donate. In a study of young African American women, the most important reason for not donating was inconvenience, followed by fear of needles and taking too much time.

A study of mailed sickle cell disease educational packets to increase blood donation within the African American community resulted in a short-term but not a long-term increase in the number of African American donors. Therefore, recruitment and retention of African American blood donors may require continual education of the African American community regarding the need for blood products, especially in the treatment of sickle cell disease patients.

My personal opinion on the matter is that people need to be enlightened, educated, get more knowledge about giving blood. I have spoken about giving blood to people, and their first response, without thinking it through, is to say no. But after taking time to explain how they would be doing something worthwhile and appreciated, which would be helping someone else within their own ethnic background, then there is a change of outlook.

The motivators for a white and black person are miles apart when it comes to giving blood. Black people cited the following reasons as barriers to giving blood, that giving blood takes too long, that the whole process can be an inconvenience and the treatment of the medical staff.

We need to educate our people more in order that they comprehend the significance, relevance and life-saving experience it is to give blood. I believe that once people understand better why they are being asked to give blood and they come forward, they similarly need to be educated that it has to be a regular thing and not just a one off wonder. The rule of thumb is that one must wait at least eight weeks to 16 weeks (56-112 days) between blood donations.

I also think one of the other factors is spirituality and fear; as they say information is key but in places of faith, blood is associated with sacrifice of some sort and as such, people are frightened to give blood because they don't know where their blood will end up. Nowadays, faith leaders and other black influencers are being spoken to about reaching out to their communities.

The Bible talks about 'life in the blood' and that is so true, to give blood is to give life to someone else, to give blood is to save a life; to give blood is to help save someone in time of need etc.

Then again, we need to keep talking about this, until it becomes second nature to us to give blood. I would like to encourage you, as you read this; if you know that you are fit and healthy; if you are age between 17-66 years old then please find time to walk into your local hospital and ask about giving blood if you can because I know for a fact that there is another ethnic minority person that you don't know who needs that blood that you are donating. Or if you live in Britain, then go online to: www.blood.co.uk

Sickle Cell and Insomnia

Sickle cell disease (SCD) is a genetic disorder that affects a protein called hemoglobin in red blood cells (RBCS), the blood cells that carry oxygen from the lungs to all the tissues in the body. The defective protein forms aggregates within the RBCs, making them stiff and giving them a sickle shape. These abnormal RBCs stick to the inner lining of small blood vessels, preventing blood low, lowering blood oxygen levels, and causing episodes of pain called vaso-occlusive crises.

People with sickle cell disease (SCD) are at an increased risk of sleep disorders as compared to their healthy counterparts. This is possibly because of disease processes, pains and living with a chronic ailment result in chronic sleep disruption that can affect developmental and health outcomes. Adequate sleep is an essential component of classic development, mood, affects regulation and health maintenance. As SCD is a chronic disease that can be affected by environmental, health, and behavioural factors, understanding the impact of the disease on fragmented sleep is important to maximize the quality of life in the lives of those living with the disorder.

A sleep expert, Dr Michael Twery in NIH said, "sleep affects almost every tissue in our bodies, it affects growth and stress hormones, our immune system, appetite, breathing, blood pressure and cardiovascular health". Research shows that lack of sleep increases the risks of infections, obesity and heart disease.

Poor sleep pattern in the lives of those with SCD risks the upsurge of developmental and psychological problems, beyond those caused by SCD itself.

Also, lack of sleep may affect the disease course, by aggravating symptoms. People with SCD are affected by sleep-disordered breath, limb movement problems, restless legs syndrome and nocturnal enuresis. Never mind, dealing with the chronic and acute pain associated with SCD, hypoxemia (oxygen deficiency in the blood), daytime tiredness and fatigue are all enough to disrupt one's sleep at night.

The effects of pain on sleep are also a significant concern, with both acute and chronic pain in SCD. SCD is associated with pain and there is no doubt it reduces sleep efficiency, slow-wave sleep and rapid eye movement sleep and shorter night sleep duration. When one has sleep disturbance, it has been related to a lower quality of life related to physical health and greater functional disability.

People's sleep quality is aggravated by SCD pain, and during a crisis, the sleep duration is even less. Ordinarily, people who experience stress find it difficult to sleep and the same is with people with SCD except that the stress is one of intense pain and this results into negative relationship with sleep.

One of the side effects of living with pain and not sleeping well is negative moods. Pain and poor health result in sleep deprivation. Most times, the vaso-occlusive crisis will start in the middle of the night. And one could associate sleep with pain and might not want to go to bed for fear of having a crisis in the middle of the night.

The impact of pain related sleep loss in the lives of people with SCD is enormous. The more the pain related discomfort is, the more the quality of one's relationship with sleep decreases; the two are intertwined.

Insufficient overnight sleep could interfere with pain-coping skills and alter the perception of pain. Due to disruptions in overnight sleep that can occur in people living with SCD may also experience more daytime sleepiness than counterparts. Also increased occurrence of sleep-disordered breathing in people with SCD can also add to higher levels of daytime sleepiness.

People with SCD experience more fatigue, due to sleeplessness at night. The connection between fatigue, sleep, quality of life and pain in the lives of people with SCD affects cognitive functioning and academic performance for sure. All of these intensified by stress, anxiety and depression.

Pain and sleep disturbance are two key elements of people with SCD. Pain disrupts sleep, which then increases the severity of pain and the risk of developing chronic pain. The result of this is patients with SCD, means less sleep at night, take more time to fall asleep and spend more time awake during the night. These have a hug impact on quality of life and overall health.

Sleep disordered breathing is of particular concern in patients with SCD as it leads to nighttime hypoxia (the body is deprived of oxygen supply). Hypoxia induces sickling in sickle RBCs.

As hypoxia is increased, risk of sickling and crisis pain is high. During the day the oxygen level with people with SCD is much higher than during the night. Living with acute or chronic pain is likely to affect one's sleep pattern negatively.

People can help by: Limit the consumption of caffeine; limit alcohol intake, treat the bedroom strictly for sleep only and not like a living room and practice relaxation techniques.

PART 8: MORE ON BENEFITS OF FOOD

Someone emailed me and asked about what food and snacks are good for people with Sickle Cell. How about eating more roasted plantain, roasted yam, ground nuts, cashew nuts, coconut, cocoyam chips, scotch eggs, beans cake, plantain chip, fruits (fresh or dried), and corn (roasted or boiled). Also form the habit of carrying a bottle of water to drink with you but nothing fizzy. I know water is bland, add some lemon or lime, mint or ginger and infuse the water as you wish.

One of the ways to safely manage SCD is to eat well. Let's look at fruits that can be eaten on the go and are healthy for us - carrot (good for eyes), banana (good for energy), orange (good source of Vitamin C), apple (good for the immune system), African cherry or Agbalumo or Udara (good source of calcium - teeth), tiger nuts or Ofio or Aya or Imumu (good for stomach constipation), Guava (good source of vitamin C), Garden eggs (good for the digestive system).

The following vegetables, meat, fish, nuts and fruits have many more nutritional value, than what I have written down.

Apple: improves digestion, prevention of stomach disorders, gallstones, constipation, liver disorders, anemia, diabetes, heart disease, rheumatism, eye disorders, a variety of cancers, and gout. It also helps in improving weakness and provides relief from dysentery. Apples also help in treating dysentery. Furthermore, they aid in dental and skin care.

The long list of health benefits attributed to apples is due to the wealth of vitamins, minerals, nutrients, and organic compounds that are found in them. These important nutritional elements include vitamin C, vitamin K, vitamin B6, and riboflavin, as well as minerals like potassium, copper, manganese, and magnesium. Apples are also very good sources of dietary fibre, and a single serving provides 12% of the daily fibre requirement. The real value of apples lies in its organic compounds. It is packed with phytonutrients and flavonoids like quercetin, epicatechin, phloridzin, and various other polyphenolic compounds.

Avocado: These days, avocado has become an incredibly popular food among health-conscious individuals. It's often referred to as a superfood, which is not surprising given its health properties. Here are some of the most abundant nutrients: **Vitamin K:** 26% of the daily value, **Folate:** 20% of the DV, **Vitamin C:** 17% of the DV, **Potassium:** 14% of the DV (DV), **Vitamin B5:** 14% of the DV, **Vitamin B6:** 13% of the DV, **Vitamin E:** 10% of the DV.

It also contains small amounts of magnesium, manganese, copper, iron, zinc, phosphorous and vitamins A, B1 (thiamine), B2 (riboflavin) and B3 (niacin).

Beans: on the whole beans are good for you and it is a meal that can be eaten in so many different ways, cooked on its own, with rice, in salads, can be dips, as a soup or blended and stuffed with other rich goodness and steamed etc.

There are variety of beans: Azuki bean; black or turtle bean (my favourite); butterbean; chick pea; cranberry bean, black eyed beans; broad bean; green bean; haricot bean.

There are also kidney bean; lentil bean; butter bean; navy bean; pinto bean; pole bean; soya bean; white bean; winged bean; asparagus bean and wax bean and more.

They are packed with protein, carbohydrates, vitamins and minerals and low in fat. In addition, beans are a good source of B vitamins (5, 6 & 12) potassium, folic acid and fibre, which promotes digestive health and relieves constipation. Eating beans may help prevent colon cancer, and reduce blood cholesterol (a leading cause of heart disease). Beans retain about 70 percent of their B vitamins (after preparation) as well as high levels of folate, which helps form red blood cells.

Each variety of beans has its own specific nutritional value, I have only concentrated on the general nutrients. If interested check out the beans institute online.

Banana: Bananas are among the most important food crops on the planet. Bananas are a healthy source of several vitamins, minerals, fibre, vitamin B6, vitamin C, and various antioxidants and phytonutrients. Bananas are a good source of potassium. A diet high in potassium can lower blood pressure in people with elevated levels and benefits heart health. Vitamin B6. Bananas are high in vitamin B6. One medium-sized banana can provide up to 33% of the Daily Value (DV) of this vitamin. Vitamin C. Like most fruit, bananas are a good source of vitamin C. Several antioxidant flavonoids are found in bananas, most notably catechins.

Cabbage: despite its impressive nutrient content, cabbage is often overlooked. Cabbage is loaded with vitamins and minerals.

If you want to improve your digestive health, fibre-rich cabbage is the way to go. This crunchy vegetable is full of gut-friendly insoluble fibre, a type of carbohydrate that can't be broken down in the intestines. Insoluble fibre helps keep the digestive system healthy by adding bulk to stools and promoting regular bowel movements.

It is rich in vitamin B6 and folate, both of which are essential for many important processes in the body, including energy metabolism and the normal functioning of the nervous system.

In addition, cabbage is high in fibre and contains powerful antioxidants, including polyphenols and sulfur compounds. Antioxidants in cabbage protect the body from damage caused by free radicals. Cabbage is especially high in vitamin C, a potent antioxidant that may protect against heart disease.

Cabbage contains vitamin C, also known as ascorbic acid, is a water-soluble vitamin that serves many important roles in the body. It's needed to make collagen, the most abundant protein in the body. This helps with the proper functioning of the bones, muscles and blood vessels.

Cabbage also contains small amounts of other micronutrients, including vitamin A, iron and riboflavin. Cabbage is a terrific source of vitamin K1, delivering 85% of the recommended daily amount in a single cup. One of its main functions is to act as a co-factor for enzymes that are responsible for clotting the blood.

Carrots: are one of the most widely used and enjoyed vegetables in the world, partly because they grow relatively easily, and are very versatile in a number of dishes and cultural cuisines.

Most of the benefits of carrots can be attributed to their beta carotene and fibre content. This root vegetable is also a good source of antioxidant agents. Furthermore, carrots are rich in vitamin A, Vitamin C, Vitamin K, vitamin B8, pantothenic acid, folate, potassium, iron, copper, and manganese.

Coconut meat (raw): The super high-fibre content acts like a probiotic, feeding the good bacteria in the intestines and keeping you regular. It's fresh juice, is rich in electrolytes, it aids in hydration, providing minerals essential for bodily functions such as movement and brain function.

Coconut is high in dietary fibre and contains a whopping 61% of fibre. Coconut helps to produce energy by burning fat. Eating coconut regularly, supports the development of healthy bones and teeth. Eating coconut regularly also helps in promoting blood circulation. Let's enjoy eating more of our coconut.

Eggs: are a very good source of inexpensive, high quality protein. More than half the protein of an egg is found in the egg white along with vitamin B2 and lower amounts of fat and cholesterol than the yolk. The whites are rich sources of selenium, vitamin D, B6, B12 and minerals such as zinc, iron and copper. Egg yolks contain more calories and fat.

They are the source of cholesterol, fat soluble vitamins A, D, E and K and lecithin – the compound that enables emulsification in recipes such as hollandaise or mayonnaise.

Some brands of egg now contain omega-3 fatty acids, depending on what the chickens have been fed (always check the box). Eggs are regarded a 'complete' source of protein as they contain all eight essential amino acids; the ones we cannot synthesise in our bodies and must obtain from our diet.

Eggs also contain more Vitamin D than they did 10 years ago, which helps to protect bones, preventing osteoporosis and rickets. And they are filling too. Eggs for breakfast could help with weight loss as the high protein content makes us feel fuller for longer. Eggs should be included as part of a varied and balanced diet.

Eggplant: Eggplants, also known as aubergines, belong to the nightshade family of plants and are used in many different dishes around the world. Eggplants are a nutrient-dense food, meaning they contain a good amount of vitamins, minerals and fibre in few calories. The fibre, potassium, vitamin C, vitamin B-6, and antioxidants in eggplants all support heart health. In addition to containing a variety of vitamins and minerals, eggplants boast a high number of antioxidants.

A serving of eggplant can provide at least 5% of a person's daily requirement of fibre, copper, manganese, B-6, and thiamine. It also contains other vitamins and minerals.

(Oily) Fish: are good for us. There is a large variety of oily fish that you can choose from: Salmon, Trout, Mackerel, Herring, Sardines, Pilchards, Kipper, Whitebait, Carp, Tuna (fresh only), Anchovies, Swordfish, Jack fish, Herring and Kippers.

As well as larger types like Ocean tuna, Atlantic salmon, Spanish various mackerels, eel, trout, silver warehouse, mullet, trevally, sand whiting and snapper.

Oily fish is very rich in omega-3 polyunsaturated fatty acids. While white fish also contains these fatty acids, levels are much lower. As well as being a super source of omega-3 oils, oily fish contains plenty of lean protein and vitamin D.

Fig: Figs and their leaves are packed with nutrients and offer a variety of potential health benefits. They may promote healthy digestion. Figs also contain small amounts of a wide variety of nutrients, but they're particularly rich in copper and vitamin B6.

Copper is a vital mineral that's involved in several bodily processes, including metabolism and energy production, as well as the formation of blood cells, connective tissues, and neurotransmitters.

Vitamin B6 is a key vitamin necessary to help your body break down dietary protein and create new proteins. It also plays an important role in brain health.

Ginger: has a long history of relieving digestive and stomach problems, as someone with Sickle Cell, this is a problem that I have, due to the strong painkillers that we take.

Ginger helps with nausea, stomach muscle pain, has anti-inflammation properties, stomach cramps, flatulence, it gets rid of throat/nose congestion, indigestion, vomiting and motion sickness and severe pain during period pains.

Grapes: the health benefits of grapes include their ability to treat constipation, indigestion, fatigue, kidney disorders, macular degeneration and the prevention of cataracts. Grapes, one of the most popular and delicious fruits, are rich sources of vitamin A, vitamin C, vitamin B6 and folate in addition to essential minerals like potassium, calcium, iron, phosphorus, magnesium and selenium.

Grapes contain flavonoids that are very powerful antioxidants, which can reduce the damage caused by free radicals and slow down aging. Grapes, due to their high nutrient content, play an important role in ensuring a healthy and active life.

Honey: it is best to take honey instead of sugar, as it can lead to long term benefits. Where honey shines is in its content of bioactive plant compounds and antioxidants. Darker types tend to be even higher in these compounds than lighter types.

High-quality honey is rich in antioxidants. Antioxidants have been linked to reduced risk of heart attacks, strokes and some types of cancer. They may also promote eye health. The antioxidants in honey may prevent free radicals from damaging the cells that line the digestive tract, which can cause acid reflux.

Honey may also be able to reduce inflammation in the esophagus and provide a coating for its mucous membrane. Again, honey is a rich source of phenols and other antioxidant compounds. Most bees deposit hydrogen peroxide into the honey as they synthesize flower pollen.

Add that honey is naturally acidic, and you have a recipe for antibacterial properties. Honey, has been shown to decrease the severity and duration of diarrhea. Honey also promotes increased potassium and water intake, which is particularly helpful when experiencing diarrhea.

Heirloom tomatoes: Heirloom tomatoes are loaded with health benefits. Tomatoes are high in fibre and a good source of vitamin A, C, B2 ... folate and chromium. The vitamins act as antioxidants, which neutralize free radicals to stop the condition of oxidative stress. Tomatoes are also rich in potassium. Heirloom tomatoes contain lycopene, one of the most powerful natural antioxidants.

Iceberg lettuce: These lettuce contain vitamin C, a powerful antioxidant that helps keep your immune system healthy. Calcium, which keeps bones and teeth strong. It also supports muscle function, nerve function, and blood clotting.

Vitamin K, a vitamin that works with calcium to prevent bone fractures. It's also integral for blood clotting. Vitamin A (as beta carotene), a powerful antioxidant that helps to maintain night vision and eye health. It also supports cell growth. Folate, a B vitamin that helps to make DNA and genetic material.

Jute leaves: are also called Lalo, Saluyot, Egyptian Spinach (Molokheya), Bush Okra, or Ewedu in West African or Sorrel depending on the region of the world. Jute plants are widely found in tropical and subtropical areas from Asia to Africa where they are mostly used in cooking. The leaves are used in stews, soups, tisanes or teas.

Other usage of Jute leaves are various health benefits because it has been determined to contain an ample amount of Vitamin A, thiamine, riboflavin, ascorbic acid, and is also rich in fibre. It is used as an anti-inflammatory treatment and a wrinkle reducer because it contains antioxidant substances

Researchers have found these plants, which are eaten as traditional foods in parts of Africa, are perhaps some of the most nutritious vegetables on the planet.

They claim jute mallow, amaranth leaves, spider plant and African nightshade contain more protein and iron than kale, which has become popular for its reputation as a superfood.

The vegetables are also rich in calcium, folate and vitamins including A, C and E according to some work.

Kale: is described as being of the cabbage family. It is quite hard raw, compared to spinach that you can have as a salad. In some food circles, it is called a super food.

Kale is low in calories but high in fibre; high in irons, high in vitamins (A, C, K and B6). Kale is filled with antioxidants and is a great anti-inflammatory food; it is also high in manganese, calcium, copper, potassium and magnesium.

Kiwi: Kiwi fruits are very low in protein and fat (0.6g each), but they are an excellent source of vitamins and minerals. Kiwi fruit is well-known for its high vitamin C content. They're also a source of some vitamin E, which helps to support the immune system.

It contains folate, the natural form of folic acid that helps the body form healthy red blood cells; calcium, a building block of healthy bones and teeth, and potassium, which supports heart health.

Lemons: Lemon water will provide your body with plenty of hydrating electrolytes in the form of potassium, calcium and magnesium. Lemon water can help reduce both joint and muscle pain. Lemon water also aids your liver in helping it release toxins. Lemon water can help cleanse your blood and arteries. Lemon water allows your body to keep a higher pH level, helping your body fight off diseases.

Mixing a teaspoon of lemon juice per half glass of water can help relieve heartburn. Drinking warm lemon water can help your body with digestion. Indigestion and constipation: Lemon juice helps to cure problems related to indigestion and constipation.

If kidney stones are a concern for you, drinking lemon water can help dissolve not only those but gallstones, pancreatic stones and calcium deposits as well.

What are the benefits of getting enough vitamin C?

It stimulates white blood cell production, vital for your immune system to function properly. As an antioxidant, vitamin C also protects cells from oxidative damage. Plus, getting enough vitamin C helps the immune system keep colds and flu at bay. Drinking lemon water daily ensures your body gets a sizable amount of vitamin C daily.

Liver: is often overlooked as an undesirable part of the bird. Liver does contain a large amount of cholesterol, but it also supplies healthy doses of many essential vitamins and minerals.

A liver provides a healthy dose of iron and zinc. Iron enables your body to use oxygen efficiently and to make new red blood cells. This mineral also plays a role in cell division and the health of your immune system. An iron deficiency can cause fatigue, decreased oxygen and a weakened immune system.

The reason why liver is one of the best superfoods and healing foods today is it's your highest source of B vitamins, iron and vitamin A. It's also a fantastic source of phosphorous and magnesium. In fact, if you compare it to spinach nutrition, carrots, an apple and some of nature's richest foods, it outperforms all of them.

The number one benefit of consuming liver is it's very high in vitamin B12, and we know vitamin B12 benefits red blood cell formation and improves cellular function; it's important for so many things. In addition to vitamin B12, liver is high in vitamin B6, biotin and folate. Those B vitamins especially folate, help your body with something called methylation as well as cellular function.

Liver also is packed with vitamin A and iron. If you struggle with any type of anemia — a clear sign of an **iron** deficiency — this is probably the best food to consume in the world because it contains folate, iron and vitamin B12. These are the three vitamins and minerals you need in order to overcome anemia naturally.

Moringa: is good for you, it boosts energy, which we tend to lack with Sickle Cell; Moringa has significant high levels of vitamins (A, B, B1,B2, B3, D, AND E); it has fibre, calcium, potassium and protein; contains anti-oxidants, rejuvenates the body cells and strengthens the immune system.

Mangoes: It also contains small amounts of phosphorus, pantothenic acid, calcium, selenium and iron. One cup (165 grams) of mango provides nearly 70% of the RDI for vitamin C — a water-soluble vitamin that aids your immune system, helps your body absorb iron and promotes growth and repair. Mango is packed with polyphenols — plant compounds that function as antioxidants. Antioxidants are important as they protect your cells against free radical damage. Free radicals are highly reactive compounds that can bind to and damage your cells.

Vitamin A is essential for a healthy immune system, as it helps fight infections. Meanwhile, not getting enough vitamin A is linked to a greater infection risk. Mango also contains folate, vitamin K, vitamin E and several B vitamins, which aid immunity as well.

For instance, it offers magnesium and potassium, which help maintain a healthy pulse and your blood vessels relax, promoting lower blood pressure levels.

Nuts: do remember that you could be allergic to some nuts or none. I know I am to some of them.

Packed with protein, fibre and essential fats. A golf ball-sized portion (about 30g) of unsalted nuts makes a vitality-boosting snack and, unlike most other options, contributes a mix of valuable vitamins and minerals.

ALMONDS: If you avoid dairy, calcium-rich almonds are a good choice to ensure you're getting enough of this bone-building mineral. Almonds are also high in vitamin E, a nutrient which helps to improve the condition and appearance of your skin.

For some extra heart help, swap flaked almonds for the whole nut – with the skin intact – because the almond's skin is full of heart-protecting compounds called flavonoids.

BRAZIL NUTS: Brazils are a good source of the mineral selenium, which we need to produce the active thyroid hormone. Selenium also supports immunity and helps wounds to heal. You only need three or four Brazil nuts a day to get all the selenium you require.

CASHEW NUTS: Cashew nuts are an excellent source of several vitamins and minerals that support healthy blood and immune system function. It has a high content of iron, zinc, phosphorus, potassium, vitamin E and B6, folic acid and manganese. The copper and iron in cashew nuts work together to help the body form and use red blood cells.

This in turn keeps blood vessels, nerves, bones and the immune system healthy and functioning properly. It's copper content, assist in energy production and provides flexibility in blood vessels, bones and joints.

Cashew nuts have a high content of magnesium which protects and supports healthy muscles and bones. We have heard that carrots are good for your eyes, you may be surprised to hear that so are cashew nuts. Cashew contain high levels of lutein and zeaxanthin, which act as antioxidants. When consumed regularly, these antioxidant compounds can protect the eyes. Cashews are protein rich and our body uses it for energy and it is particularly important for rebuilding muscle tissue and creating new cellular compounds.

CHESTNUTS: By far the nut with the lowest fat and calories. Chestnuts are rich in starchy carbs and fibre, and in their raw form are a good source of vitamin C.

They're lower in protein than other nuts but make a useful contribution of B vitamins including B6. Ground chestnut flour can be used as a gluten-free flour for cakes and bakes, or buy fresh and roast for a tasty snack.

MACADAMIAS: Although high in fat, they do supply good levels of the healthy mono-unsaturated variety. They're a rich source of fibre and make a useful contribution of minerals including magnesium, calcium and potassium.

PEANUTS/GROUNDNUTS: They are rich in vitamins and minerals and contain 13 different types of vitamins, they include vitamins A, B, C & E. They are also rich in 26 essential minerals including, calcium, iron, zinc, etc… all these help to strengthen the bones and purify the blood.

They are known to combat depression and help blood related problems in women. Lastly, they have a high concentration of anti-oxidants.

PECANS: Heart-friendly pecans are packed with plant sterols, valuable compounds that are effective at lowering cholesterol levels. Pecans are also antioxidant-rich which helps prevent the plaque formation that causes hardening of the arteries. They're rich in oleic acid, the healthy fat found in olives and avocado. As a good source of vitamin B3 pecans are the perfect option if you're fighting fatigue because this vitamin helps us access the energy in our food.

PISTACHIOS: Being especially rich in vitamin B6, which is important for keeping hormones balanced and healthy, pistachios are a good option for those with problem periods.

They're the only nut to contain reasonable levels of lutein and zeaxanthin, two antioxidants that play an important role in protecting the eyes. Pistachios also contain potassium and fibre – in fact a 30g serving has more than three times that supplied by the equivalent weight of plums.

WALNUTS: Their superior antioxidant content means walnuts are useful in the fight against cancer. They're also a good source of mono-unsaturated, heart-friendly fats, and studies show they help to lower the bad form of cholesterol (LDL). Finally, they're rich in omega-3, so they're a great alternative if you don't eat oily fish.

Okra: Who would have thought that Okra is very good for people with Sickle Cell? Yes it is! It is also referred to as 'lady's fingers' or 'gumbo'.

The rich fibre and mucous like content in the Okra pods helps ease digested food and constipation conditions. The pods contains vitamin (A, B complex, C and K) as well as a high amount of anti-oxidants.

The consumption of food rich in vitamin C helps the body develop immunity against infections, reduced episodes of colds and cough and lastly protects the body from harmful free radicals. The pods equally contain good minerals such as iron, calcium, magnesium and manganese.

Onion: Onions have several health benefits, mostly due to their high content of antioxidants and sulfur-containing compounds. They have antioxidant and anti-inflammatory effects and have been linked to a reduced risk of cancer, lower blood sugar levels, and improved bone health.

Folate (B9), a water-soluble B vitamin, folate is essential for cell growth and metabolism and especially important for pregnant women.

Vitamin B6 is found in most foods, this vitamin is involved in the formation of red blood cells. Potassium, this essential mineral can have blood pressure-lowering effects and is important for heart health. Onions contain decent amounts of several vitamins and minerals, including, Vitamin C, an antioxidant, this vitamin is needed for immune function and maintenance of skin and hair.

Pawpaw or papaya: the fruit is extremely rich in vitamin C which help in keeping your cells healthy and your immune system strong. It is also rich in vitamin A, which helps your vision from degenerating.

They are good for your bones, as they have anti-inflammatory properties. It has a digestive enzyme known as papain along with fibre which helps improve your digestive health. It's a rich source of minerals, namely magnesium, potassium and iron. Eating pawpaw, helps your body metabolize the other foods you eat. It contains vitamins B6, riboflavin, folate, niacin and thiamin. These B complex vitamins work together to help your body convert protein, carbohydrate and fat into energy. Pawpaw also contains anti-oxidants.

Plantain: is rich in fibre and adequate amount of dietary-fibre in the food helps normal bowel movements, thereby reducing constipation problems. Fresh plantain have more vitamin C than bananas.

Consumption of foods rich in vitamin-C helps the body develop resistance against infectious agents and scavenge harmful oxygen-free radicals.

The most abundant nutrient in plantains is carbohydrate. Plantains carry more vitamin A than bananas. Besides being a powerful antioxidant, vitamin A plays a vital role in the visual cycle, maintaining healthy mucus membranes, and enhancing skin complexion.

As in bananas, they too are rich sources of B-complex vitamins, particularly high in vitamin-B6 (pyridoxine). Pyridoxine is an important B-complex vitamin that has a beneficial role in the treatment of neuritis, anemia, and to decrease *homocystine* (one of the causative factors for stroke episodes) levels in the body. In addition, the fruit contains moderate levels of folates, niacin, riboflavin and thiamin.

They also provide adequate levels of minerals such as iron, magnesium, and phosphorous. Magnesium is essential for bone strengthening and has a cardiac-protective role as well.

Fresh plantains have more potassium than bananas. Potassium is an important component of cell and body fluids that helps control heart rate and blood pressure, countering negative effects of sodium.

Quail eggs (QE): should be classified as a supper food. Despite its small size, its nutritional value is 3-4 times more than that of a chicken egg. It is not known to cause allergies of any kind.

QE are generally rich in anti-oxidants, in protein and iron. QE is a source of vitamins (A, B1, B2, B6, B12 and D), copper, zinc, magnesium, and other mineral and amino acids. It strengthens the immune system and help with anemia by increasing the level of hemoglobin in the body while removing toxins.

Red cabbage: it tastes similar to green cabbage. However, the purple variety is richer in beneficial plant compounds that have been linked to health benefits, such as stronger bones and a healthier heart. It is rich in vitamins C and K.

Red cabbage has a good mix of vitamins and minerals, especially folate, which is essential during pregnancy and also helps the body to produce red blood cells. It also contains vitamin C, which helps protect our cells by acting as an antioxidant, and potassium. Anthocyanins are antioxidants that are found in purple-coloured fruits and vegetables, including red cabbage.

Raspberry: One cup of raspberries provides over 50% of the minimum daily target for vitamin C, which supports immunity and skin health and helps produce collagen. Raspberries also contain manganese and vitamin K, which both play a role in bone health. And they supply smaller amounts of vitamin E, B vitamins, magnesium, copper, iron, and potassium.

Spinach: this leafy green is another 'super food' and classified as one of the world's healthiest food, loaded with nutrients and has small calories, so good to eat.

It is rich in iron, contains protein, minerals and vitamins (A, B1, B2, B6, C, E, K) and folic acid. It also contains calcium, potassium, manganese, magnesium, zinc etc...It is known to add vitality, improve the quality of the blood and repair energy.

Strawberries: are an excellent source of vitamins C and K as well as providing a good dose of fibre, folic acid, manganese and potassium. They also contain significant amounts of phytonutrients and flavanoids which makes strawberries bright red.

They have been used throughout history in a medicinal context to help with digestive ailments, teeth whitening and skin irritations. Their fibre and fructose content may help regulate blood sugar levels by slowing digestion and the fibre is thought to have a satiating effect. Leaves can be eaten raw, cooked or used to make tea.

Tripe: seems like an unconventional choice compared to more common diet staples like chicken breast, drumsticks, wings, lamb, steak etc... it's worth adding to your diet. Tripe is relatively low in calories, it serves as a source of essential nutrients that benefit your health. Tripe serves as a source of minerals as well as protein and vitamins your body relies on for good health.

Tripe is high in Vitamin B-12 and contributes to your daily vitamin B-12 intake. Getting enough vitamin B-12 benefits circulation and also proves important for nervous system health. It promotes red blood cell function by helping to make a protein that these cells need to transport oxygen.

It contains vitamin B-12, which is only naturally found in significant amounts in animal products; B 12 is important for forming DNA and red blood cells to carry oxygen throughout your body.

Turmeric: is high in iron, which is good for warriors. It is also high in vitamins, (E, B6 and C). It contains lots of minerals for example, manganese, copper, calcium, iron, potassium and it's got anti-inflammatory content.

Remember, turmeric is difficult to wash off when it spills, either on clothes or work surfaces, so do be careful as you pour it.

Veal: is a nutritious powerhouse because of the following – Selenium, this meat also contains elements like selenium. Selenium helps protect the system against free radicals, which provokes cardiovascular diseases and cancers.

Iron: The human body needs iron in red blood cells to transport oxygen. Iron is a great source of energy too. Vitamin B12: This vitamin helps a lot for our energy and it also helps for the red blood cells reproduction. Vitamin D: also known as the "sunshine vitamin", contributes to a proper functioning of muscles and bone health.

Phosphorus: This metalloid is omnipresent in our system and helps for bone metabolism, neurological system and energy. Magnesium fights depression. Zinc is excellent against cold, flu, as well as some digestive problems. Vitamin B3 has got plenty of benefits.

Wheat: is probably the most common cereal available all over the world and is in even higher demand in recent years due to its abundant health benefits. Foods like bread, pasta, crackers, bagels, cakes, and muffins are just a few common examples of wheat sources.

Whole wheat is also a major source of dietary fibre, which the bowels need to work properly, as is important in the life of someone with Sickle Cell.

Wheat is rich in catalytic elements, mineral salts, calcium, magnesium, potassium, sulphur, chlorine, arsenic, silicon, manganese, zinc, iodide, copper, vitamin B, and vitamin E. This wealth of nutrients is why wheat is often used as a cultural base or foundation of nourishment.

Watermelon: Drinking water is an important way to keep your body hydrated. Interestingly, watermelon is 92% water. Watermelon has many other nutrients as well, including these vitamins and minerals: Vitamin C, is an antioxidant that helps prevent cell damage from free radicals. Vitamin A, Potassium, Magnesium, Vitamins B1, B5 and B6.

Watermelon is also high in carotenoids, including beta-carotene and Lycopene. This potent antioxidant gives a red color to plant foods such as tomatoes and watermelon and is linked to many health benefits. Plus, it has citrulline, an important amino acid.

Yam: contains vitamins (A, C, D, E, K, B6, B12 and more). Contains anti-oxidants, carbohydrates, minerals, such as (Calcium, Iron, Magnesium, Potassium, Zinc and Copper).

Yams are not only an excellent source of fibre but also high in potassium and manganese, which are important for supporting bone health, growth.

These tubers also provide decent amounts of other micronutrients, such as copper and vitamin C. Copper is vital for red blood cell production and iron absorption, while vitamin C is a strong antioxidant that can boost your immune system.

Yellow squash: The vegetable is high in vitamins A, B6, and C, folate, magnesium, fibre, riboflavin, phosphorus, and potassium. That's a serious nutritional power-packed veggie.

Yellow squash is also rich in manganese. This mineral helps to boost bone strength and helps the body's ability to process fats and carbohydrates.

Savor the color and texture of this brightly hued veggie by lightly braising it to create smothered yellow squash with basil.

My personal daily drink/snack

In a nutshell, here are some of the benefits of a drink that I have daily. I use: *Hibiscus leaves*: packed with anti-oxidants, good supply of iron and B-vitamins. *Mint leaves*: relieves indigestion, has immune boosting benefits and treats nausea. *Moringa*: Rich in iron, vitamins (B6, B1, B2, A, and C) and packed with anti-oxidants. *Ginger*: treats nausea and soothes digestive system, contains vitamin B6 and helps in pain reduction. *Beetroots*: great source of fibre, contains folate (vitamin B6), contains vitamins A and C and it is rich in iron.

Lemons: good source of vitamin C and contains anti-oxidants, helps with digestion. *Cloves*: contains vitamins K, E and C; is a good source of fibre and has anti-oxidant properties. *Star anise*: it is rich in anti-oxidants, helps to treat digestive ailments such as bloating, gas, indigestion and constipation. *Juniper berries*: helps increase the flow of urine, a good source of vitamin C and rich in anti-oxidants. *Tumeric:* contains powerful medicinal properties; increases anti-oxidant capacity in the body; has benefits against depression amongst other benefits.

I clean and cut all the above in small pieces, add honey or sugar cane sugar and infuse in hot water and leave to infuse for a few hours (3-6). After which, I pour in bottles, put them in the fridge and drink a glass a day.

If you want to drink the above as a smoothie, you can cut in pieces and pulse in your liquidizer.

I eat nuts: (cashew, peanuts and hazelnuts) and these also contain vitamin E. I am trying to now eat eggs regularly and vegetables because of their vitamin B6 content.

Chicken, turkey, pork meant and fish also contain vitamin B6. You also need vitamin B12 and you can find these in beef, chicken, fish, eggs, liver, low fat milk and cheese.

You can also get more vitamin C from sweet and white potatoes, green and red peppers and tomatoes. Most of these food also contain zinc, which is good for you.

I'm also into cooking vegetable soups, the one thing I do, is mix vegetables and not just cook Ugu for example. I will most probably mix other green leaves with Ugu, namely spinach or kale and others; a lot of these greens contain vitamin E and C, which is necessary for someone with Sickle cell.

CONCLUSION

I hope you have enjoyed reading this book and learning more about SCD.

The important thing about self-care is eating well. This will help other areas of your life too. Your body will respond positively to you not putting junk inside it and your outlook about life will be positive.

You will have a confident attitude to life and your energy levels will be boosted because your physical and mental states are robust too. As your mood becomes more upbeat, you will start living and stop existing.

I tend to bang on about healthy eating because for every tablet I take, that is related to Sickle cell, there will be some negative side effects in my body and I don't like that. I would rather, eat something prepared at home, as I take the tablets and not eat biscuit; drink my self-made drink or water, instead of some bottled, fizzy or carton drink, that have preservatives and other things in them, to make them last for a week, two weeks or a month and more.

Dear warrior, don't let Sickle Cell stop you from living your life to the full; don't look at yourself but instead aim high and go for what you want to achieve in life. No one can stop you from becoming what you want to become except you. Surprise yourself and you will be pleasantly astonished as you achieve your goals in life.

REFERENCES

www.acidalkalinediet.net

www.arthritis.org

www.bbc.co.uk

www.beaninstitute.com

www.bloodjournal.org/

www.bmj.com

www.caribbeangreenliving.com

/www.cdc.gov

www.clevelandclinic.org

www.counselling.uk

www.davidwolfe.com

www.draxe.com

www.evelinalondon.nhs.uk/

www.fitday.com

www.food.gov.uk

www.foodwatch.com.au

www.gpnotebook.co.uk;

www.guysandstthomas.nhs.uk

www.havesttotable.co.uk

www.healthline.org

www.health.usnews.com

www.heart.com

www.helpguide.com

www.hematology.org

www.huffingtonpost.com.au

www.lebonheur.org

www.lifespan.org

www.livescience.com

www.mayoclinic.com

www.medicalnewstoday.com

www.medlineplus.gov

www.medscape.com

www.mind.org.uk

www.nature.com

www.ncbi.nlm.nih.gov

www.newsinhealth.nih.gov

www.ncbi.com

www.nhlbi.nih.gov

www.nhs.co.uk

www.onhealth.com

www.oatext.com

www.onlinelibrary.wiley.com

www.organicfacts.net

www.pennstatehershey.adam.com

www.premierhealth.com

www.primarypsychiatry.com

www.sciencedaily.com

www.sicklecellanemianews.com

www.sickle.bwh.harvard.edu

www.sicklecellsociety.org

www.sleepfoundation.org

www.stjude.org

www.tescoliving.com

www.thelancet.com

www.uptodate.com

www.vitastiq.com

www.wedmb.com

www.weforum.org

www.weightwatchers.com

www.wellnessmama.com

www.whfoodscom

ABOUT THE AUTHOR

A little bit more about me, I have worked in the media industry for over twenty years and worked for the best media company in the world, the BBC. Of course, I would fall ill from time to time but never once thought not to work and stay at home because of Sickle Cell.

I make sure that Sickle Cell does not define me but I define Sickle Cell. By that I mean people find it hard to believe that I have Sickle Cell, until I fall ill, in a very bad way. People with Sickle Cell, you know what I am talking about or if you know someone with Sickle Cell, then you know too. Let's live as best as we can by eating ourselves to wellness.

I am a relationship counsellor and a coach.

I write as a columnist (on a weekly basis) on issues pertaining to SCD, for the Nigerian newspaper Punch.

I am an author, my books are sold in paperback and kindle format on Amazon and okada books.

I am also a blogger:

www.howtolivewithsicklecell.co.uk

www.howtohaveacareerinyour40sandbeyond.co.uk

 www.pastors1stlady.co.uk

Printed in Great Britain
by Amazon